607 ESSENTIAL OIL USES

FOR HEALTH AND HEALING, FOR BEAUTY, FOR PETS, FOR HOUSE, FOR OUTSIDE AND FOR FOOD.

SAMANTHA K. RAY

This document is geared towards providing exact and reliable information in regards to the topic and issue covered. The publication is sold with the idea that the publisher is not required to render accounting, officially permitted, or otherwise, qualified services. If advice is necessary, legal or professional, a practiced individual in the profession should be ordered.

- From a Declaration of Principles which was accepted and approved equally by a Committee of the American Bar Association and a Committee of Publishers and Associations.

The information provided herein is stated to be truthful and consistent, in that any liability, in terms of inattention or otherwise, by any usage or abuse of any policies, processes, or directions contained within is the solitary and utter responsibility of the recipient reader. Under no circumstances will any legal responsibility or blame be held against the publisher for any reparation, damages, or monetary loss due to the information herein, either directly or indirectly.

The information herein is offered for informational purposes solely, and is universal as so. The presentation of the information is without contract or any type of guarantee assurance.

TABLE OF CONTENTS

INTRODUCTION

I want to thank you and congratulate you for downloading the book, *"607 Essential Oil Uses"*.

This book contains essential oil uses for health and healing, for beauty, for pets, for house, for outside and for food.

I will take you in a journey through the essential oil uses so that you understand them better and learn how to use them.

Thanks again for downloading this book, I hope you enjoy it!

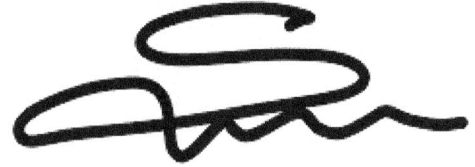

Samantha K. Ray

DISCLAIMER

None of the health benefits or claims that are included in the following text have been approved or evaluated by the FDA. As with all things you should make sure that you use your own judgment or contact a health care professional for concerns that you might have. The following is not meant to treat, cure, prevent, or diagnose any disease. These benefits are for symptom relief and general health maintenance and require that you use all natural 100% organic essential oils that are pure to get the mentioned benefits.

A Few Notes on Therapeutic Grade Oils

When it comes to using essential oils it is important that you know what you are using. Make sure that you purchase therapeutic grade oils in order to be able to gain these health benefits. If you do not have the right oils you might even find yourself having adverse issues from using the oils.

Here are the reasons that it is important to purchase therapeutic grade oils:

- They use the proper plant varieties.

- The plants that produce the oils are grown in indigenous regions around the world.

- The plants that are used for the oils are grown without any chemicals of any kind. No pesticides are used with these plants.

- The harvesting is done at peak times to make sure that you get all of the properties and benefits of the oil.

- The extraction is done at temperatures and pressures that help to ensure the oil molecules are not damaged.

- The therapeutic companies will stand behind the internal use of their products.

- The companies pay for third party testing of each and every batch of oils that they produce.

Keep in mind that you should never take an essential oil internally if it is not therapeutic grade.

Tea Tree Oil and melaleuca Tree Oil Uses

Tee tree oil and melaleuca tree oil can be used in many of the same ways. Just replace melaleuca tree oil for the tee tree oil for all of the following benefits.

Precautions: Tea Tree Oil should not be taken internally as it can be toxic when ingested.

Keeping tea tree oil in your medicine cabinet is a great idea. The following are 80 different ways that you can use tea tree oil in your home.

For Health and Healing

1.   Abrasions and Minor Cuts:

You can place tea tree oil on minor cuts and abrasions once they have been cleaned. It may be necessary to dilute the tea tree oil in a base oil.

2.   Acne:

Applying tea tree oil directly to the acne is an effective treatment that is completely natural. You can leave this treatment on your skin overnight. Some people find that the oil by itself is a little too harsh and find that they like the results of mixing it with a carrier or oil or even into their regular face wash.

3.   Allergies:

Massaging tea tree oil that has been diluted in a carrier oil on the chest and reflex points on the feet can help reduce allergies.

4.   Arthritis

Those suffering from arthritis can find relief but putting twenty drops of tea tree oil into two ounces their carrier oil of choice. They can massage this on the affected parts of their body for instant relief.

5. Asthma:

One of the best ways to treat asthma with tea tree oil is to put a few drops into a pot of water. Then bring this to a boil, remove the water from the stove, and drape a towel over your head breathing in the vapors. This should quickly clear your head and help relieve symptoms of as asthma.

6. Athlete's Foot:

Applying tea tree oil lighting to your feet with a cotton ball two or three times each day can help the infection to disappear. For someone who has sensitive feet or sores from the athlete's foot, they can dilute ten drops of the oil in 1 tablespoon of carrier oil.

7. Baby Care:

There are many things that you can do with tea tree oil with babies. Spraying diaper pails with a mixture of tea tree oil and water can keep them clean. Using five drops of tea tree oil that has been mixed with two tablespoons of coconut oil and quickly and naturally take care of diaper rash.

8. Bacterial Infections:

Adding a few drops of tea tree oil to a bath or massaging onto the affected area can quickly clear up bacterial infections.

9. Bad Breath:

Bad breath can be cured with one drop of tea tree oil that has been mixed with one ounce of water. Just swish in your mouth like you would mouthwash and spit out.

10. Bladder Infections:

Sitting in a bath that has between ten and fifteen drops of tea tree oil can quickly help relieve the symptoms of a bladder infection.

11. Blisters:

Adding a drop or two of tea tree oil to a blister that has been cleaned can help it clear up and heel quickly.

12. Boils:

Before applying tea tree oil to a boil, use a warm washcloth and hold it on the boil for a couple of minutes. Next apply a drop to the area. The inflection will quickly rise to the surface where it can be released.

13. Bronchial Congestion:

Use in the same way that you would for bronchitis.

14. Bronchitis:

Follow the instructions for asthma and then add ten drops of the oil to one ounce of a carrier oil to massage onto the chest and throat two or three times each day.

15. Bruises:

Apply ice to the area first and then follow up with the oil in the same manner as that used for arthritis.

16. Bunions:

Massage the area with five drops of tea tree oil that has been diluted with one tablespoon of carrier oil.

17. Burns:

Rinse the area with cool water for ten minutes. Next wait a few minutes while the area air dries a bit. Wait a few minutes and apply a mixture of 5 drops of tea tree oil and one teaspoon of honey. Reapply this to the area between three and five times until it has healed.

18. Calluses/Corns:

Use five drops of oil in one tablespoon of a carrier oil and massage the area three times each day. When the area has softened you can remove excess skin and treat the area with the oil directly applied and then a bandage placed over it.

19. Canker Sores:

Use a cotton swab dipped in tea tree oil to treat the area two times each day. You can also use the same method as what is used for bad breath.

20. Carbuncles:

Use a cotton swab to apply a drop of the oil to the carbuncle three times each day.

21. Chapped Lips:

Use one drop of tea tree oil in coconut oil and use on your lips when they feel really cracked, sore, or dry.

22. Chicken Pox:

Use a drop of the oil on the blisters, allow the oil to dry, and then dust with corn starch. This can be repeated every few hours until the blisters are healed.

23. Chigger Bites:

While it might sting, applying the tea tree oil to the chigger bites will quickly get rid of them.

24. Cold Sores:

Add tea tree oil directly to the cold sores with a cotton swap three to four times per day.

25. Coughs:

Use the same methods as what are used for bronchitis.

26. Dandruff:

To quickly get rid of dandruff just add ten drops of tea tree oil to every 8 oz of shampoo that you already use. Shake the bottle well to make sure that it has been evenly distributed into the shampoo. You can also massage tea tree oil directly onto your scalp.

27. Dermatitis:

Put ten drops of tea tree oil into one tablespoon of carrier oil and use this to massage onto the areas that are affected three or four times per day.

28. Dry Skin:

Gently rub a mixture of five drops of tea tree oil and one tablespoon of sweet almond oil onto the skin.

29. Earache/Ear Infection:

Mix together three drops of tea tree oil and two tablespoons of warm olive oil. Use a dropper to drip a few drops into the ear and tilt head to the side to clean up an excess oil. You can repeat this two or three times each day.

30. Eczema:

Adding ten drops of tea tree oil to a carrier oil and massaging on to the affected areas of the skin three or four times each day can help to heal the areas.

31. Emphysema:

Do the same steps as bronchitis.

32. Flea Bites:

Apply a drop of oil directly to the bites.

33. Gout:

Massage a mixture of two tablespoons of carrier oil and ten drops of tea tree oil on the area two or three times each day.

34. Gum Disease / Homemade Mouthwash:

Use purified water, one drop of peppermint oil, and one drop of tea tree oil to make your own mouthwash. Swish this around in your mouth two or three times each day for thirty seconds and spit it out.

35. Head Lice:

Use twenty drops of oil in two tablespoons of shampoo and massage on the scalp and hair. Leave this mixture on the hair for at least ten minutes. Rinse and repeat three or four times each day until there are no eggs left.

36. Hives:

Mix ten drops of tea tree oil with four tablespoons of witch hazel and apply to the infected areas. Alternate this mixture with ten drops of tea tree oil and four tablespoons of coconut oil for sensitive skin.

37.   Immune System:

Boost your immune system by spraying a mixture of tea tree oil and water or diffusing tea tree oil throughout your home. You can also massage the oil on the soles of your feet to increase you immune system.

38.   Infected Wounds:

Add tea tree oil to steaming water and hold the wound over the stem. In addition you can combine one drop of tea tree oil and one cup of water to pour over the infected area one or two times each day until healed. You can also try spraying the mixture on the wound if it is too painful to pour the water over it.

39.   Inflammation:

Use a diffuser to diffuse and breath tea tree oil or massage tea tree oil over inflamed areas in a rubbing motion towards your heart.

40.   Ingrown Hairs:

Simply put a drop or two of oil on the ingrown hair every two hours until the infection is gone.

41.   Jock Itch:

Mix together between ten and fifteen drops of tea tree oil and two tablespoons of a carrier oil and then apply twice daily. Allow to dry and dust with corn starch.

42.   Laryngitis:

Make a mixture of five to ten drops of tea tree oil, a pinch of sea salt, and one cup of warm water to gargle between two and three times each day.

43.   Mosquito Bites:

Apply a drop of tea tree oil to the bite.

44.   Muscle Aches and Pains:

Draw a warm bath and add in one half of a cup of Epsom salts and between ten and fifteen drops of oil. Allow this to dissolve. After having taken a bath massage sore muscles with ten drops of tea tree oil that has been diluted in two tablespoons of a carrier oil.

45.   Mumps:

Use tea tree oil to massage all over the body and the feet while diffusing it throughout your home.

46.   Nail Fungus:

Paint tee tree oil directly onto affected nails two times each day for a time period of two months.

47.   Planter Warts:

Apply one or two drops to the wart between two and three times a day until it is no longer present.

48.   Psoriasis:

Mix together ten drops of tea tree oil and one tablespoon of carrier oil to massage onto affected skin three or four times each day.

49.   Rashes:

Mix together coconut oil and tea tree oil to massage gently over the rash.

50.   Rheumatism:

You can mix together twenty drops of tea tree oil to two ounces of carrier oil to massage onto areas that have been affected by pain.

51. Ringworm:

Put one or two drops of tea tree oil directly onto the ringworm three times each day. You can add a drop of lavender oil for some added benefits.

52. Rubella:

Mix together tea tree oil and a carrier oil to massage onto affected areas. Diffuse lemon oil, tea tree oil, and lavender oil to keep the infection from spreading.

53. Scabies:

Add one or two drops of tea tree oil to affected areas every morning and every night.

54. Sciatica:

Mix together one tablespoon of a carrier oil with ten drops of tea tree oil and use this two or three times each day to massage the area.

55. Seborrhea:

For the skin you can mix ten drops of tea tree oil with one tablespoon of carrier oil to be massaged onto the area three or four times each day. For the scalp you can mix ten drops of tea tree oil with your favorite shampoo and massage on hair allowing ti to sit on the scalp for ten minutes before rinsing between four and five times each day. You can also add between ten and fifteen drops of tea tree oil to your bath.

56. Shingles:

Add ten to fifteen drops of tea tree oil and half of a cup of Epsom salts to the bath and dissolve. You can also mix together two tablespoons of coconut oil or grapeseed oil with ten drops of tea tree oil to massage onto the shingles.

57.   Shock:

Massage tea tree oil onto the souls of the feet as often as needed to reduce the risk of shock.

58.   Sinusitis:

Use ten drops of tea tree oil in a steamer to be used for between five and ten minutes. You can also add one or two drops to a neti pot before use.

59.   Sore Throat:

Do the same thing that you would for Laryngitis.

60.   Staph Infection:

Follow the steps for immune support.

61.   Stye:

Put five drops of tea tree oil to a pot of water that is steaming. Drape a towel over your head and allow this to steam your face for five minutes. When finished apply a warm compress to the eye.

62.   Sunburn:

Mix together one tablespoon of coconut oil with one drop of lavender oil and one drop of tea tree oil to carefully apply to the sunburn.

63.   Tattoos:

After you have gotten a tattoo you can reduce the chances of getting an infection by applying tea tree oil that has been diluted with coconut oil or spray on a mixture of tea tree oil and purified water.

64. Thrush:

Mix together warm water, one drop of tea tree oil and sea sat and gargle.

65. Ticks:

If you get bitten by a tick place a few drops of tea tree oil onto a cotton ball and hold the cotton ball on the tick for one minute. Do this until the tick can easily be removed with a pair of tweezers. Then apply a drop of oil to the bite to make sure that you do not get an infection.

66. Toenail Fungus:

Put tea tree oil on the infected nail and underneath the tip of the nail. Apply two drops of the tea tree oil to the nail at bedtime.

67. Tonsillitis:

Follow the steps for laryngitis and for bronchitis.

68. Vaginal Infection:

You can add a few drops of tea tree oil to your bath or you can add one drop of tea tree oil to one tablespoon of carrier oil and coat a tampon with it. After you have coated the tampon you can insert it and leave it in place for a day. If there is irritation you should immediately remove the tampon and wash the area with clean and warm water.

69. Viral Infections:

Diffuse tea tree oil throughout your house and inhale from hot steaming water.

70.   Warts:

Apply tea tree oil directly to the wart repeating both morning and night until the wart is gone.

IN YOUR HOUSE

71.   Air Freshener:

Using a diffuser to disperse the oils or putting tea tree oil on a cotton ball and placing in a small open container in a room is a safe and effective way to get rid of bad odors. This option is perfect for keeping your home natural.

72.   Toothbrush Cleaner:

Put one or two drops of tea tree oil onto your toothbrush two times each week to kill all of the lingering bacteria.

73.   Pest Control:

Most household bugs like ants do not like tea tree oil. Putting drops of the oil into doorways can be a cost effective way to deal with pests. In addition you can create a mixture of water and tea tree oil to clean cabinets and counter tops with.

74.   Laundry Helper:

You can prevent mold by adding one to two teaspoons of tea tree oil to you laundry.

75.   Mildew and Mold Remover:

You can combine two teaspoons of tee tree oil and two cups of water in a bottle. Shake well and then spray onto mold and mildew. Then letting it dry without rinsing.

76.   Insect Repellant:

Mix together 15 drops of tea tree oil and a quarter cup of water in a spray bottle to be sprayed all over your body and clothes.

77.   Household Cleaning:

Use tea tree oil to make your own cleaners that sanitize surfaces and get rid of germs. A great easy recipe for a tea tree oil cleanser is to mix two teaspoons of tea tree oil and two cups of water in a spray bottle and shaking this to mix well.

78.   Flea Collar for Dogs:

You can make your own flea collar for your dogs by applying a few drops of diluted tea tree oil to their colors. Make sure that you are using a carrier oil and that is very well diluted so that it does not affect your dog's skin.

79.   Carpet Cleaning:

Adding a few drops of the oil to your vacuum bag will not only make it smell great but will also help to better clean the carpets.

Lemon Oil Uses

There are a wide variety of uses for lemon oil. Lemon oil can be used for a variety of purposes including those concerning health and healing, inside the home, outdoors, and even an addition to your food and water.

For Health and Healing

80. Sore Throat:

To soothe a sore throat add 2-3 drops of lemon essential oil to hot tea or warm water with honey.

81. Colds, Coughs, and Congestion:

If you are feeling congested you can rub lemon oil on your chest or throat multiple times throughout the day or you can diffuse it into the air.

82. Runny Nose:

It is possible to use a little bit of carrier oil and a drop of lemon oil and then to swipe this on each side of your nose to stop a runny nose.

83. Hay Fever and Allergies:

Putting a drop of lemon oil under the nose and behind the ear two or three times each day will help with allergies, as will applying to the soles of your feet.

84. Energy:

If you need a boost in energy grab your water bottle and add a few drops of lemon and peppermint oil to help you perk up.

85. Bad Breath:

Putting 4 drops of lemon oil into 4 ounces of warm water and gargling it will get rid of your bad breath.

86. Acne:

If you want to treat acne all you have to do is add three drops of lemon oil to a cotton ball and put it on the affected area three times a day or less.

87. Fatigue:

For everyone who is suffering from fatigue you can moisten a wash cloth with five drops of lemon oil and put it under your nose for two minutes long

88. Stress:

You can add ten to fifteen drops of lemon oil to your bath water for a soak that is at least fifteen minutes long and you will feel instant stress relief.

89. Minor Wounds:

Treating minor wounds can be done with lemon essential oil since it is an antiseptic. You can put five drops of lemon oil in three ounces of water in a bowl and use a sterile cloth that has been dipped in the mixture to wipe the wound. You will want to do this until the wound looks clean.

90. Corns, Callouses, and Warts:

To make the callouses, warts, and corns disappear just put a drop of lemon oil on them two times each day.

91. Canker Sores:

You can heal canker sores by adding one drop of lemon oil to a shot glass of water and swishing it in your mouth.

92. Fever Blisters and Cold Sores:

Putting a drop of lemon oil on cores and fever blisters two or three times each day will make them go away.

93. Psoriasis:

You can control psoriasis by using a roller ball that has lemon oil and coconut oil in it to put the mixture on the affected areas.

94. Nail Fungus:

With just a few drops of lemon oil on the affected nail multiple times each day you can clear up nail fungus in a few months. It is important to continue to use the oil until the fungus has completely cleared.

95. Skin:

You can brighten your dull complexion if you just add a drop of lemon oil to your moisturizer each day. Just remember to follow this with some sunscreen because you are going to increase your sensitivity to the sun.

96. Mental Clarity:

It is also possible to be more clear with your thoughts if you are diffusing lemon oil. This is great for work spaces and study spaces.

IN YOUR HOUSE

97. Make Your Toothbrush More Sanitary:

If you need to sanitize your toothbrush you should just put a drop of lemon oil on it and swish in a glass of water.

98. Clean Glass:

If you want to clean glass you can add lemon oil to a spray bottle that has been filled with water. It is also great to clean soap scum and hard water off of glass shower doors.

99. Clean the Toilets:

You can also clean toilets by adding a few drops of lemon oil with baking soda to get them both cleaned and completely sanitized.

100. Disinfect the Kitchen:

Rubbing lemon oil onto kitchen counters and cutting boards will completely disinfect them.

101. Rid Your House of Germs:

You can quickly kill germs on household rags and kitchen wash cloths by soaking them in a bowl of water that has just one or two drops of lemon oil added.

102. Have Fresh Smelling Air:

To make yourself an air freshener you can either diffuse 8 drops of lemon oil or you can add a few drops to a spray bottle that has been filled with water.

103. Get Odors Our:

You can also get rid of stubborn odors with lemon oil. All you have to do is put a few drops on a cotton ball and put it in the area where the odor is at.

104. Laundry:

If you are making your own laundry soap you can add a few drops of lemon oil the soap and if you are using store bought soap you can add a few drops to the rinse cycle so that your washer is left smelling great.

105. Get Rid of Grease:

If you have grease left on your hands or dishes you can quickly remove it with lemon oil. Lemon oil will also help you to get rid of glue, label residue, or tree sap.

106. Polish Wood:

Adding a few drops of lemon oil to olive oil that will keep furniture polished and looking great.

OUTSIDE

107. Get Rid of Mosquitoes:

Mixing lemon oil with a carrier oil and rubbing it onto your skin will keep mosquitoes away.

108. Insect Bites:

Applying two drops of lemon oil to an insect bite and lightly rubbing a few times a day will help the bite to heal quicker.

109. Sanitize Your Hands:

If you have used a public restroom or are at the park, all you have to do to have sanitized hands is to rub a drop of lemon oil on them. This also works great for kids since there is no alcohol or chemicals.

WITH FOOD AND WATER

110. Water:

You can quickly improve the taste of water and make it more enjoyable when you add a few drops of lemon oil.

111. Flavor:

Lemon oil can be added to bland foods to liven them up a bit.

112. Help Food Last Longer:

Fresh produce will last longer when you are able to put the produce into a bowl that has been filled with cold water and adding two or three drops of lemon oil.

REMEDIES USING ESSENTIAL OILS

There is a vast array of ailments that you can cure with essential oil based remedies. The following are some of the ailments that can be cured with oils that were not mentioned above.

112. Hiccups:

Just put a few drops of peppermint oil on each side of your spinal cord and on your neck.

113. Drowsiness:

If you are feeling drowsy you can be less drowsy by combining peppermint oil and wild orange oil and putting it on the back of your neck. Then you can smell your hands and inhale the leftover oil. Plus you can add four drops to a diffuser.

114. Eyes that are Itchy or Irritated:

Just put a few drops of lavender oil on the bones that are surrounding your eyes but be careful to not let the oil get into your eyes.

115. Cellulite:

If you want to get rid of cellulite then all you have to do is take 4 ounces of fractionated coconut oil and pour a bottle of grapefruit oil into it. You can rub this onto your problem areas after you get out of the shower or bath.

116. Diaper Rash:

If you are worried about diaper rash all you have to is mix together a spray with 18 ounces of water, 1 teaspoon organic body wash, 4 drops of melaleuca, and 4 drops of lavender. This always works as a great combination to prevent diaper rash as well.

117. For Your Dog with an Ear Infection:

Many people do not realize how common ear infections in dogs really are. To treat your dog quickly and naturally put one drop of melaleuca and a carrier oil on a cotton ball to wipe out the inside of their ear several times each day.

118. For Your Dog with a Sunburned Nose:

Just dab a little bit of lavender oil mixed with a carrier oil on the dog's nose for relief.

119. Fevers:

If you have a fever, add a few drops of peppermint oil that has been mixed with a carrier oil and apply it the torso and spine. This can drop the body temperature up to 3 degrees in just a few minutes.

120. Heartburn:

All you have to do to get rid of heartburn is add a few drops of peppermint oil to a small glass of milk. You can also rub a blend of oils on your chest and belly that have been made for digestion like Digest.

Coconut Oil Uses

There are also a wide array of uses for coconut oil. Here are 126 common coconut oil uses.

For Health and Healing

121. Fungal Infections:

The fatty acids that are present in coconut oil will insert themselves into the fungal membrane and will eliminate the fungus' ability to maintain life through the destruction of this membrane.

122. Care for Wounds:

Coconut oil has anti-fungal properties which makes it perfect for putting on small scratches and scrapes. Of course you do not want to put it on a large wound but it is perfect for small wounds as a natural form of first aid.

123. Diaper Rash Ointment:

Coconut oil makes the perfect diaper rash ointment for your little one.

124. Aromatherapy:

To be able to get the benefits of aromatherapy. All you have to do is make sure that you can add essential oils to the coconut oil and rub them on your temples.

125. Soothe Bee Stings:

When you get stung by a bee, coconut oil is a great way to reduce the pain, heat, and swelling that come along with it.

126. Take Care of a Chapped Nose:

If your child has a runny nose that has become chapped then you can put coconut oil on it to soothe and moisturize it.

127. Relieve the Pain from Arthritis:

Since inflammation is the main cause of pain with arthritis, coconut oil can get rid of some of the pain on its own but if you add in essential oils you will see even more benefits. You just do this two times each day.

128. Treat Athlete's Foot:

If you want to be able to get rid of athlete's foot then you should try the anti fungal properties of coconut oil. Just make sure that you are washing your hands well after application to keep from spreading the fungus.

129. Get Rid of Hangnails:

Hangnails can be painful and irritating. You can get prevent hangnails by applying coconut oil to the cuticles to prevent hangnails.

130. Treat Your Sore Throat:

Sore throats can be very painful and coconut oil is a great natural coating to soothe the pain and discomfort that you might feel. You will just need to swallow between one half and one teaspoon of coconut oil three times each day.

131. Improving Circulation:

To be able to heal problems that occur because of circulation you can massage the coconut oil to improve blood flow.

132. Reduce Osteoporosis:

There are many ways in which coconut oil can help to improve conditions that are associated with osteoporosis. Coconut oil will help to increase bone volume. Coconut oil is also great as an anti-oxidant which can help to make the bones absorb more calcium.

133. Relief from Food Poisoning:

Each year there are more strains of bacteria and germs which means that you have more of a chance of getting food poisoning. To reduce the symptoms that are associated with food poisoning you can take two or three tablespoons of coconut oil with orange juice each day. This is going to help you to get healthier faster.

134. Reduce Teething Pain:

When children are going through teething between six and nine months of age. Using coconut oil and rubbing it on the gums can help to reduce inflammation and irritation.

135. Heal Tattoos:

If you have a new tattoo you can help it to heal quickly and to stay moisturized by using coconut oil. Plus with all of the anti-inflammatory and antiseptic properties you are less likely to get an infection.

136. Add to Baby Bath:

Adding coconut oil to the bath water is going to help keep your baby's skin soft, smooth and healthy.

137. Ringworm:

Ringworm is a parasite that is much like athlete's foot and is caused by several types of mold that feed on the tissue. You need to wash your hands and then apply coconut oil to the area, careful to wash your hands afterward.

138. Psoriasis and Eczema:

Both eczema or psoriasis can be uncomfortable and can be helped by applying patches of coconut oil to the areas.

139. Dandruff:

Some people suffer from chronic dandruff because of a fungus that is on the scalp. To be able to change this you can apply coconut oil two or three times each week to be able to stop the itching.

140. Heartburn:

When you are having issues with heartburn you can quickly swallow one or two teaspoons of coconut oil. This is going to coat your stomach and will ease the pain that you have from heartburn and even acid reflux.

141. Bruises:

Bruises will heal quicker when taken internally. It will help reduce the amount of time that it takes bruises to fad or heal.

142. Acne:

Coconut oil will also help to fight acne by reducing the bacteria that causes it. If you add in a few drops of tea tree oil you will get additional acne fighting benefits.

143. Oil Pulling (for your teeth):

Oil pulling has recently become very popular. Oil pulling is said to have a number of benefits from preventing and slowing down further tooth decay to helping boost your immune system. Pulling with coconut oil is going to help you to have the most benefits. All you do is put a few teaspoons in your mouth and you swish and pull the oil through your teeth. Continue doing this for a time period of ten to twenty minutes and then spit into the trash can. Do not spit this in the sink. When you are finished rinse your mouth with a water that has been mixed with sea salt.

144. Cradle Cap:

While cradle cap is a harmless condition, using coconut oil on the affected area can help it to be less bothersome.

145. Sleep:

You can sleep better or help your loved ones sleep better when you use coconut oil as a carrier oil with lavender and other essential oils that are used for sleep and relaxation. Just rub the oil with the essential oils on your chest and the bottoms of the feet.

146. Cancer:

You can fight your risk of cancer by using coconut oil. Since coconut oil has been to have an anti-tumor affect and to help maintain your immune system it is thought that coconut oil can help to prevent cancer.

147. Yeast and Candida:

Both yeast and candida can wreak havoc on your life and your well being. You can get rid of yeast infections by applying coconut oil directly to the affected area. You can keep candida from wreaking havoc on your body and immune system by ingesting a teaspoon of coconut oil each day.

148. Balance Hormones:

The adrenal glands and thyroid are naturally balanced when the cortisol in the body is lowered. Two of the things that coconut oil does are that it suppresses inflammation and supports metabolism. Both of these are necessary for you to be able to have balanced hormones.

149. Blood Sugar:

In a 2009 study it was found that coconut oil was able to help control blood sugar levels and because it helps to regulate the amount of insulin that is secreted by the pancreas. Therefore it can be used as a treatment for prevention of diabetes.

150. Cholesterol:

You can naturally lower your cholesterol with coconut oil. This is because the fats in coconut oil have been proven to raise the good HDL cholesterol while lowering the bad LDL cholesterol. In a study done by Harvard Medical School the coconut oil was found to improve the cholesterol ratio.

151. Get Rid of a Dry Cough:

Having a dry cough can be very bothersome but with coconut oil you can take care of it. All you have to do is swallow a teaspoon of coconut oil to get instant relief.

152. Cleaning Retainers:

Coconut oil can also be used to clean a retainer after rinsing it by just rubbing the oil on and rinsing it off. You can also use coconut oil as a mouthwash to help reduce germs and bacteria on your retainer or mouth piece.

153. Cold Sores:

Cold sores are caused by the Herpes simplex virus so it is not something that can easily be cured. You can inhibit the virus from being able to spread. Just apply coconut oil to the cold sore directly a few times each day.

154. Dry Nose:

If you are going through one of those days where your nose feels dry and you feel like it needs to be picked at then all you to do is dab coconut oil on the outside and inside of each nostril. It will help your nose to heal and no longer feel as dry.

155. Relief of Constipation:

Taking a tablespoon of coconut oil on an empty stomach each morning will help you to get your digestive track in shape. If you are having more severe problems then you can try two tablespoons of coconut oil.

156. Lower Your Risk of Heart Disease:

Just by eating 1/2-1 teaspoon of coconut oil each day you can drastically lower your risk of heart disease while lowering your cholesterol.

157. Lower Your Risk of Alzheimer's:

Taking just two teaspoons of coconut oil each day can help to improve your cognitive health. This can help to lower your risk or Alzheimer's or reduce the effects of this devastating disease if you have already been diagnosed.

158. Nipple Cream:

Anyone who has ever spent time breastfeeding is going to know the pain that it can cause. Using coconut cream as a nipple cream is soothing and can help relieve all of this pain.

159. Sooth Rashes:

Coconut oil has anti-inflammatory properties so it is a perfect soother for the coconut oil. Plus it will keep you from scratching your skin.

160. As a Carrier Oil:

Coconut oil makes the best carrier oil for using essential oils. It can also be used as a base oil for sugar scrubs, massage oils, lotions, body butters, and lip balms.

161. A Vapor Rub:

To be able to make your own vapor rub all you have to do is mix together coconut oil with peppermint essential oil. Then you just apply this to your chest and your nose.

162. Reduce Your Risk of Getting Head Lice:

Head lice hates coconut oil so if you are worried about your child getting head lice than all you need to do is use a fine toothed comb to run it through your hair.

163. Inflammation:

One of the great things about coconut oil is that it is great for helping to remedy inflammation.

FOR BEAUTY

164. Skin Moisturizer:

One of the best things about coconut oil is that you can use it as a natural moisturizer for your skin. Not only does coconut oil help you by offering skin soothing relief but it also will help to heal dry skin by penetrating deep within. It might feel oily at first so it is a good idea to use this sparingly.

165. Fight Frizz:

Putting a small amount of coconut oil on your hair can help you with dryness or with keeping humidity at bay.

166. Reduce Age Spots and Sun Spots:

Using coconut oil on your sun spots, age spots, and many other skin blemishes will help them to fade away quickly.

167. Make Toothpaste Better:

You can even create your own toothpaste by using baking soda and coconut oil together. Just add in a few drops of cinnamon or peppermint oil to make it taste better.

168. Prevention of Stretch Marks:

Coconut oil can help you to prevent stretch marks by keeping skin well moisturized which can aid when it is stretching during pregnancy or growth.

169. Personal Lubrication:

Coconut oil is not compatible with latex but it is one of the best personal lubricants that you can find.

170. Detangling Solution:

You can easily use coconut oil as a great detangling solution.

171. As a Beard or Mustache Wax:

A little bit of coconut oil works as a beard and mustache wax works well.

172. Highlight Your Cheeks:

If you apply a small amount of coconut oil to your cheekbones then you are going to make them have a beautiful natural glow.

173. Get Cleaner Makeup Brushes:

Makeup brushes are made from delicate materials that break down and are ruined over time when you are cleaning them. Using coconut oil to clean them will help them last longer. Just melt some coconut oil and dip the brushes into the liquid and then swirl it on a wash cloth until it is cold. Rinse with warm water and dry.

174. Give Yourself Long Thick Eyelashes:

Instead of using mascara, you can enhance your eyelashes naturally. Applying coconut oil to your lashes does several things. It helps your eyelashes to grow naturally. It also helps to seal moisture into them and prevents breakage.

175. Tinted Lip Balm:

You can also create your own healthier tinted lip balm or even a lipstick using coconut oil. Just use the lip balm recipe and when the coconut oil is melted you can add in beet root powder, cocoa powder, cinnamon, turmeric, or any other spice that has a color that you would find flattering on your lips. Adding spices like cayenne pepper will help to plump the lips but some people find this to be an uncomfortable feeling.

176. In Grown Hairs:

You can both treat and prevent ingrown hairs with coconut oil. All you have to do is rub the areas that are prone to bumps or in grown hairs with coconut oil. There are two reasons that this works...one is that it helps the skin to be softer so that the hair can more easily grow and the other is that it naturally helps to kill bacteria.

177. Shampoo:

You can mix coconut oil with apple cider vinegar to use as a shampoo. Not only does this naturally help to wash the hair but it also helps to keep it shiny, smooth and comfortable.

178. Hair Brushes:

You can naturally clean your hair brush to remove unwanted hair that has gotten caught in the brush while also killing bacteria. It can also help to restore delicate bristles that are on the brushes. The best part is that any leftover oil will help make your hair healthier and will help with detangling.

179. Create More Lather:

You can add coconut oil to things like homemade shampoo or soap this will help to create lather that you might not otherwise be able to create without chemicals.

180. Hair Styling:

Hair styling is also made easier with coconut oil. You can use coconut oil like a mouse, gel, or texturizer. The coconut oil will also help to work as a smoother and de-frizzer.

181. Fat:

That's right coconut oil, even though it is an oil, can help to fight fat in your body. Coconut oil has been proven to help fight fat and help you to lose weight. When you take one tablespoon of coconut oil daily you will find that the fat in your body is burned quicker for energy. While it might sound odd to add a fat to your diet to burn more fat this is something that has been proven to burn stubborn abdominal fat according to the *Journal of Clinical Nutrition.*

182. Cracked Heels:

Coconut oil can also be put on cracked heels.

183. Get Rid of Split Ends:

You can prevent and get rid of split ends by applying coconut oil to the ends of your hair each day. You will be amazed by how quickly you have nice smooth hair.

184. Sun Care:

While coconut oil only provides a small amount of SPF (around 4 to 6), it is a great way to keep sunscreen active in between applications and can hydrate your skin. You will also be able to use it if you get burned.

185. Get Rid of Scalp Flakes:

Rubbing coconut oil on a dry and itchy scalp can really help to reduce the amount of flakes that you might have.

186. Get Rid of Fine Lines:

Coconut oil is a great natural skin moisturize that will help prevent fine lines and wrinkles. It will also help to increase the collagen in your skin which can actually reduce the appearance of fine lines and wrinkles that you might already have.

187. Get Rid of Your Under Eye Bags:

It is easy to get rid of your under eye bags by rubbing a little bit of coconut oil onto them.

188. To Soften Dry Elbows:

You can easily use coconut oil to moisturize and take care of your dry elbows as well.

189. Conditioner:

Coconut oil can be used as a conditioner to smooth the hair shafts and will really help on the ends of the hair where it can get the most dry.

190. Homemade Soap:

Coconut oil is the perfect base for making homemade soap. It is a wonderful and pure natural ingredient that will add harness to soap and help break down oils and grease. Plus it will keep skin from drying out. To make a great soap all you really need is a combination of lye, water, and coconut oil.

191. Weight Loss:

While you will not lose weight by just eating coconut oil there are many things that coconut can be used as in order to aid you in your weight loss journey. You can easily get rid of calories from other fats by using coconut oil instead of other oils. It is metabolized differently and it can be used as an appetite suppressant. Plus it can help you with cravings for foods that are worse for you.

192. Lip Balm:

One of the great things about coconut oil is that it can be used to n the lips as lip balm. Not only is it great for moisturizing the lips and for adding SPF protection.

193. Body Scrub:

Coconut oil is also a great base for body washes and facial scrubs. This can be done in a few different ways. One of the easiest is to melt it down and to stir in some sugar. Then all you have to is let it cool before using it. After you rinse this off you can use some coconut oil as a moisturizer.

194. Removing Make Up:

Coconut oil is also a great choice as a makeup remover. All you have to do is put it on your face and rub it in a gentle circular motion over your make. This actually works perfectly with waterproof eye makeup too. Then all you have to do is rinse your face and pat it dry. If your face still feels oily, you can use a gentle facial cleanser to clean it completely.

195. As a Massage Oil:

There are so many benefits to having regular massages. Instead of using the traditional massage oils you can use coconut oil.

196. To Treat Nails and Cuticles:

Using coconut oil to repair chipped or broken nails is something that you should do on a regular basis. This is going to quickly make your nails look perfect.

197. Shaving Cream:

Coconut oil is great to be used as a shaving cream. This can help you to make sure that you do not damage your skin during the process of shaving.

198. Soap Scum:

You can quickly apply a thin layer of coconut to soap scum. All you have to do to get rid of the soap scum is let this sit for between 10 and 20 minutes before quickly wiping it away with the rough side of the sponge.

199. Deodorant:

Mixing one tablespoon of arrowroot powder with three to four tablespoons of coconut oil is an easy way to make a homemade deodorant that is going to really work at keeping you smelling fresh.

200. As a Bath Oil:

You can also easily soften your bath water and improve the health of your skin when you add coconut oil to the water.

201. Energy Booster:

Coconut oil will give you a boost in energy. Plus it can boost mental clarity and alertness.

FOR PETS

202. Dogs that Itch:

Many dogs suffer from allergies and atopic dermatitis. Feeding your dog a tablespoon or two of coconut oil is a great way to help them reduce many skin ailments and allergies.

203. No More Hair Balls:

If you are worried about hair balls you can reduce them by rubbing coconut oil on your cat's paws. This is going to reduce the amount of hair balls and improve your cat's digestive functions.

204. As a Dog Treat:

When it is hot and during the summer you are going to be able to make treats for your dog out of coconut oil. All you need to do is mix coconut oil and peanut butter and put it into an ice cube tray and freeze it. This is a great special treat for your favorite dog. You want to make sure that you do not give these to your dog on carpeting though.

205. Cracked Dog Paws:

If your dog has cracked or dry paws then you should rub some coconut oil onto them to heal them.

206. Soothe Udders:

If you have a cow you can treat the udders by using coconut oil.

207. Make Your Dog's Coat Shine:

All you have to do is feed 1 tablespoon to dogs that weight over thirty pounds or 2 teaspoons to dogs that weigh under thirty pounds and it will improve their dry skin and give their coat a generous and beautiful shine.

208. Horse Hair:

If you have a horse, then coconut oil will work great as a mane and tail conditioner. It will help to give your horse that luxurious look that you desire.

IN YOUR HOUSE

209. Wood Polish:

You can avoid chemicals when you use coconut oil to polish your wood. It will keep it looking healthy longer and will help it keep its natural finish.

210. Polish for Leather:

To be able to polish your furniture with coconut oil you need to first dust the furniture with a dry cloth. Then you use a very small amount of coconut oil to polish the leather and make it shine.

211. Lubricant:

Coconut oil can be used as a lubricant for small motors. Remember that you just want to use a little bit and that melted generally will be the best form.

212. Get Rid of Insects:

Using coconut oil with essential oils (citrus and peppermint are great choices) is a great weary to make your own natural bug repellant. Insects seem to hate coconut oil.

213. Make Your Eggs Last Longer:

If you have eggs you can make them last longer by being able to paint the eggshell with a thin layer of coconut oil.

214. Ink:

Have you ever had ink smear all over your hands? Instead of trying to scrub it off, just rub some coconut oil on and let it set for a few minutes before wiping it off with a clean dry cloth.

215. Get Rid of Rust:

All things that are metal are going to eventual rust from being exposed to oxygen. If you want to get rid of rust all you have to do is spread a thin layer of coconut oil on the rusty spots. You just have to let it stand for one or two hours rand then run warm water over them while wiping clean with a soft polishing cloth.

216. Remove Stains from Tupperware:

Tupperware can easily be stained with different sauces and things. Instead of worrying about stains, treat your Tupperware with a thin layer of coconut oil that you let allow to dry and soak into the plastic. This is going to treat it and protect against future stains.

217. Car Detailing:

You can use coconut oil to detail your car and buff out small scratches from your paint.

218. Stuck or Squeaky Hinges:

If you have a squeaky door or a door that is stuck then you can apply coconut oil to the hinges. It will help them not to stick or be squeaky.

219. Candles:

You can also use coconut oil as a carrier oil for candles. Instead of burning candles with chemicals and harmful materials in them you can burn the oil by itself and diffuse with essential oils. This is better for you and your family.

220. Shoes:

Coconut oil can be rubbed onto leather shoes and synthetic leather shoes to make them shine.

221. Removing Gum:

Coconut oil does a great job at removing chewed gum from hair and carpeting.

222. For Your Cast Iron Pans:

If you have a cast iron pan and you need to season it then using coconut oil and generously rubbing it into the pan before putting the pan in an oven that has been heated to 250-350 degrees for an hour is going to help perfectly season the pan.

223. Conditioning a Cutting Board:

All you have to condition a cutting board is wipe it with a damp towel and dry it completely. Then you have to use a soft cloth to rub the coconut oil and let it stand for ten to fifteen minutes.

224. Polish Metal:

Using coconut oil with a soft cloth is a great way to rub on metal to buff them and make them shine.

225. Get Rid of Dust:

Rubbing a thin layer of coconut oil on wood or dashboards of car is going to repel and keep dust from collecting.

226. Make Plants Shine:

To give plants a beautiful dust free shine then you just need to rub a small amount of coconut oil onto the leaves. You can easily reapply this every few days to keep the leaves shiny.

227. Lawn Mower Maintenance:

Apply a thin layer of coconut oil to a clean lawn mower blade will prevent grass clumps from sticking to it and causing jams in the mower.

228. Bicycle Chains:

You can easily grease your bicycle chains with a thin layer of coconut oil on them.

229. Kitchen Appliances:

You can rub thin layer of coconut oil over the blades on kitchen appliances. This will help to keep them running smooth.

230. Get Help with Your Snow Shoveling:

You can clear snow easily by applying coconut oil to your shovel. It can be reapplied as needed and you can use it to keep the snow from sticking to your shovel.

231. Get Rid of Tree Sap:

Rubbing coconut oil on your hands or clothes when they have gotten tree sap on them will make the sticky mess go away.

232. Stuck Zipper:

If you have a stuck zipper then you should check out coconut oil and whether or not it can help the zipper to glide with ease.

OUTSIDE

233. Fly Bites:

Coconut oil works well at soothing painful fly bites. This is great for people as well as for pets.

FOR USE WITH FOOD

234. Frying and Sauteing:

One of the reasons that coconut oil is so great for sauteing and frying things is that hit has a high smoke point which means that you are able to choose an oil with healthier fats that is safe too.

235. Buttering:

You can use coconut oil in the same way that you would use butter in "buttering" things.

236. Energy Boosting:

Mixing one tablespoon of coconut oil with one half tablespoon of chia seeds will give you a great snack that is packed full of what you need for energy. You can spread this on a grainy bread or an apple or you can eat it by itself.

237. Coffee:

Use coconut oil in replace of cream and sugar. If you put your coffee into a blender with the coconut oil you can create any number of amazing coffee drinks without adding unnecessary and unhealthy sugars.

238. Fondue:

If you love dipping fresh fruit into dark chocolate you make it even healthier with the addition of coconut oil. Just mix together one tablespoon of coconut oil and two cups of chopped dark chocolate for a delicious fruit dip that you are sure to love.

239. Smoothies:

You can make fruit smoothies healthier with the addition of one or two tablespoons of coconut oil. As an added bonus the flavor will be improved and you can reduce the amount of sugar or sweetener that you add to it.

240. Popcorn:

Cooking your popcorn in coconut oil and then using it to drizzle on the popcorn with some sea salt.

241. Replace Cooking Spray:

You can use coconut oil for everything that you would have used cooking spray for. Plus it helps make clean up easier.

242. Healthier Homemade Mayonnaise:

Making a healthier mayonnaise is easy when you use coconut oil. The easiest recipe is to take 4 egg yolks, 1 tablespoon of apple cider vinegar, and ½ teaspoon of dried mustard and mix them together in a blender. While the blender was running you can slowly add in 1 cup of melted coconut oil and ½ cup of olive oil mixed together very slowly so that you do not have the mayonnaise break.

243. Sweet Potatoes:

Adding coconut oil to baked sweet potatoes with some cinnamon is a delicious way to enjoy this special treat. You can even bake them in the oven to make fries with rosemary and sea salt.

244. Baking:

You can replace butter and other oils with coconut oil. When you are using it in place of butter in baked goods you need to use 70% coconut oil and 30% water to get the same amount. If you do not do this you will not have the right texture. You also can use the coconut oil to grease pans and baking dishes.

245. Granola:

Using coconut oil to make your own homemade granola for breakfast or a snack can really help you to stick to a heart healthy diet while eating something delicious. You can even top your own Greek yogurt and fruit parfaits with the granola that you make. To make granola you need to combine 3 cups of old fashioned oats, 2 teaspoons of cinnamon, 1 cup of chopped almonds, ½ teaspoon of salt, 1/3 cup coconut palm sugar with ½ cup honey. Melt 1/3 cup coconut oil and drizzle this over the above mixture and then bake at 350 for 5-7 minutes. Rotate it in the oven and then bake for another 5-7 minutes. Turn the oven off and allow to sit in the oven for an additional 30 minutes. After this you can remove from the oven and break it into pieces.

246. Sports Drink:

Many people try to boost their energy with processed sports drinks but instead you can add coconut oil and chia seeds to the water that has fresh fruit in it for flavor.

PEPPERMINT OIL USES

Peppermint oil is known for its many benefits and its ability to help you in a number of different ways. Peppermint oil is another must have for anyone who wants to try and be more natural and even for those who do not. The benefits from this essential oil are amazing.

PEPPERMINT OIL BENEFITS

- Get rid of stomach aches

- Freshen your breath

- Get rid of headaches

- Help yourself to focus

- Have a clear respiratory tract

- Boost energy

- Release tight muscles

- Replace many pharmaceutical medications

FOR HEALTH AND HEALING

247. Pain Relief for Sore Muscles:

When you have sore muscles peppermint oil is one of the best natural pain relievers and muscle relaxers that you can find. Some users even feel like it works better than the pharmaceutical drugs that they might have taken for years. Peppermint oil can be helpful on many different parts of the body but seems to really help with sore backs, painfully sore muscles, and tension headaches. One study even showed that people suffering from fibromyalgia pain and mysofascial pain syndrome were able to find relief with peppermint oil.

248. Sinuses:

Diffusing peppermint oil into the air and inhaling it can help to instantly make it easier to breathe. It will clear your sinuses and help to relieve itchy throats tat the same time. It is a great treatment for coughs, asthma, colds, bronchitis, and sinusitis. When trying to control congestion you can massage a few drops of peppermint oil that has been added to a carrier oil into the chest. You can also add a drop to the humidifier. Plus if you are feeling like your head is extra stopped up you can create your own peppermint steam to breath by making a pot of boiling water and adding peppermint oil to it. Then stand with your head over the steam and drape a towel over you. Take deep slow breaths to get the maximum benefit.

249. Joints:

If you have achy joints you can apply pure peppermint oil that has been combined with lavender oil to the achy areas. Doing this will cool your muscles much like an ice bath so it is important to make sure that you stay dry and warm.

250. Allergies:

One of the great benefits of peppermint oil is that it can help to relax the muscles that are in your nasal passage. It can also help you to clear out pollen and other allergens. If you suffer from allergies, try diffusing peppermint oil with eucalyptus oil and clove oil for maximum relief.

251. ADHD:

To help your child with being able to stay alert and focusing you can either spray some peppermint oil on their shirt before study time or have them place a drop of peppermint oil under their tongue.

252.   Itch Relief:

You can apply a mixture of peppermint oil and lavender oil to a rash or any type of itchy skin for cooling and healing relief.

253.   Reduce Fevers:

One of the best benefits of peppermint oil is that it can be used to naturally bring down fevers. This is especially beneficial in children. All you have to do is mix peppermint oil with coconut oil and then rub it on your child's neck and the bottom of their feet to control fevers the natural way.

254.   Acne:

Since peppermint contains anti-microbial properties it is effective in helping to naturally cure acne.

255.   Headaches:

Peppermint oil will help to relieve headaches by improving circulation, healing the stomach, and relaxing tense muscles. Migraines and tension headaches can be relieved by applying peppermint oil to the temples and forehead. Peppermint oil can be used to help relieve a number of additional symptoms including sensitivity to light and noise.

256.   Get Rid of Nausea:

Peppermint oil was found to reduce nausea that has been induced by chemotherapy better than medical treatments in one recent study. To get the benefits you can add one drop of peppermint oil to water and drink or you can diffuse peppermint oil or even put one or two drops of the oil behind your ears.

257. Respiratory Problems:

You can open up your airways naturally with peppermint oil. It can be used as a decongestant or mixed together with coconut oil and eucalyptus as a homemade vapor rub. Peppermint oil has been shown to reduce the symptoms that are associated with bronchitis and asthma.

258. Colic:

In a recent study medical researches discovered that using peppermint oil on infants with colic was just as effective as the medication Simethione which has a number of concerning side effects. With peppermint oil there are no side effects.

259. Teething:

Peppermint oil is also a great choice for helping to relieve teething pain in infants. All you have to do is mix peppermint oil and coconut oil in equal amounts and rub this mixture on the baby's gums for instant relief.

260. Stress Relief:

Peppermint oil is one of the essential oils that has been known to have benefits for those who are suffering from stress, mental exhaustion, and even depression. This is because is naturally refreshing and invigorating. It can also help you to feel less restless and anxious. If you are trying to relieve stress a great combination to try is peppermint oil, lavender oil, and geranium oil in a bath. This will help to relieve stiffness in the muscles and body that are often associated with stress as well as being absorbed into the skin to help you to internally relax. Using aromatherapy with a diffuser and peppermint oil can also help to reduce stress.

261. Bug Bites:

Using a combination of peppermint and lavender oil on bug bites is going to make the itchiness go away completely. You will want to dilute this with a carrier oil if you are sensitive and it could sting or a burn a bit otherwise.

262. Heartburn:

To get rid of heartburn you can add a drop or two of peppermint oil to your tea along with a teaspoon of honey. You can also add a drop or two of peppermint oil to a glass of milk. Plus you can add five drops of peppermint oil to a teaspoon of coconut oil and massage this into your stomach.

263. Feeling Drowsy?:

If you are feeling drowsy you can combine peppermint oil with lemon or orange oil and apply this to the back your neck. When you are done with this you can inhale the leftover that is on your hands.

264. Constipation:

If you are struggling with constipation then you can combine peppermint oil with a carrier oil to be massaged into your lower abdomen. This will help to get things going in the right direction and can keep you regular.

265. Remove a Tick:

To remove a tick you can soak a q tip in peppermint oil and dab this on the tick. When the tick withdraws its head you can easily remove it.

266. Painful Tendons:

If you are experiencing painful tendons you can mix together ten drops of peppermint oil, ten drops of lavender oil, ten drops of rosemary oil, and two tablespoons of a carrier oil. You can massage this in the areas that are sore and you will find that your pain seems to melt away.

267. Craving Control:

Inhaling peppermint essential oil will help keep your cravings controlled. It will also help you to feel full faster. One great thing to do is use peppermint oil in a diffuser during meal times. Another is to simply put a couple of drops on your temples or chest before eating. You can also just breathe in the scent from the bottle.

268. Boost Energy:

Energy drinks are dangerous and some have even been proven to contain toxic ingredients. If you want to perk yourself up without these harmful drinks then you can just smell peppermint oil. This is great for when you are on long car trips or when you are going to need to be able to stay awake and alert longer. It can also help someone who has been diagnosed with chronic fatigue syndrome to be able to concentrate and focus better. To instantly improve your concentration you can simply rub a drop of peppermint oil under your nose. This will make you feel energized and alert. If you are struggling with energy throughout the day you can apply the peppermint oil to your neck and shoulders throughout the day. Doing this repeatedly will help to energize you even when you have not been able to sleep or are feeling exhausted and worn out. Additionally before working out you can inhale peppermint oil and instantly get a boost in your energy levels which can help you to work out harder and longer.

FOR BEAUTY

269. Shampoo:

One great thing that you can do to help yourself wake up during your morning shower is to add two or three drops of peppermint oil to your regular shampoo. This will provide a tingling and energizing sensation to your scalp which can help you to wake up quickly. It is also a great antiseptic so it can help to remove dandruff and lice as well as help prevent against lice naturally without the chemicals that commercial products might contain.

270. Healthier Teeth and Fresher Breath:

Peppermint has been used for over 1000 years to naturally freshen breath. In fact many commercial breath fresheners use peppermint oil. Peppermint oil has been proven in studies to do a better job at reducing cavities than the chemicals that are found in mouthwash. You can make your own mouth wash and tooth paste. You can also put a drop of peppermint oil under your tongue and drink a glass of water for fresher breath.

271. Sore Feet:

If you have sore feet that are tired and aching then you can add a few drops of peppermint oil to a foot bath. This will really help you to have some relief while reducing swelling.

272. Skin Problems:

Peppermint oil will help with skin inflammation. It can be mixed into lip balm to help heal cracked lips and to sooth sore lips in the winter months. It can also be added to body lotion to get the same effects on skin problems. Using peppermint and lavender together and also improve eczema and psoriasis.

273. Hair:

Peppermint oil has been used for quite some time in some of the most high end hair care products. The reason for this is simple because it can help to nourish damaged hair while helping to make the hair thicker. You can make your own homemade shampoo with peppermint oil or add a few drops of peppermint oil to your favorite shampoo to help combat hair loss and help promote hair growth.

274. Sunburns:

You can also use peppermint oil to hydrate skin that has been sunburn as well as to relieve pain. Just mix a few drops of peppermint oil into some coconut oil.

275. IBS:

For IBS you can actually take peppermint oil internally in a capsule form. In a recent study 75% of participants saw a 50% reduction in their IBS symptoms when taking peppermint oil on a regular basis.

276. Indigestion and Bloating:

One of the great things about peppermint oil is that it can be taken to reduce colon spasms because it relaxes your intestines. This can also help to reduce gas and bloating. You can drink peppermint tea or add one drop of peppermint oil to your water before meals in order to see these benefits. To get these benefits there are some additional things that you can do as well. You can massage a few drops of peppermint oil on your stomach and abdomen or place a drop on your wrists. You can also inhale if you feel like you will be sick. Drinking peppermint tea can also be helpful and is easy to make at home.

277. Weight Loss:

Peppermint oil can help you to lose weight. When you inhale peppermint oil it is a natural appetite suppressant.

IN YOUR HOUSE

278.   Repel Pests:

Ants, ticks, mosquitoes, spiders, lice, mice, and cockroaches all hate peppermint oil. Using peppermint oil in a diffuser or just making your own natural floor cleaner with peppermint oil can help to keep these pests away.

279.   Trash:

For stinky trash you can add a few drops of peppermint oil to the bottom of the trash can which will leave a nice minty aroma

280.   Air Freshener:

To freshen the air in your home add peppermint oil to a diffuser.

281.   Clean Your Home:

There are many ways that you can clean your home with peppermint oil. Mixing together ½ cup of white vinegar, 32 ounces of water, and ½ teaspoon of peppermint oil can make a great multi-purpose cleaner for your home.

EUCALYPTUS OIL USES

There are many great ways in which eucalyptus oil can help to heal ailments that might be weighing you down or causing problems in your life.

FOR HEALTH AND HEALING

282. Arterial Vasodilator:

Eucalyptus oil has been show to help increase circulation by helping to dilate the circulatory system. You can easily massage one drop on any area where you might want to improve circulation.

283. Asthma:

If you have an asthma attack you can massage one or two drops of eucalyptus oil onto the chest. You can also inhale the aroma from the bottle or diffuse eucalyptus oil into the air.

284. Brain Health:

Eucalyptus oil can be used to help improve blood flow to the brain. This can be done by diffusing and is perfect for times when you are trying to study or in a classroom setting.

285. Bronchitis:

You can use eucalyptus oil to massage into the chest, back, and/or throat. You can also inhale from the bottom or add a drop to your shirt collar or diffuse to help clear up bronchitis.

286. Congestion:

You can clear congestion from the airways and nasal passages by inhaling eucalyptus oil and massaging it on the affected areas.

287. Temperature Control:

You can use eucalyptus to cool your body down. This is perfect for the summer or after a work out. The best way to get these benefits it put five to ten drops of eucalyptus oil and five to ten drops of peppermint oil into a spray bottle and fill it with water.

288. Coughs:

Eucalyptus oil can help to get rid of coughs when it is diffused into the room. It can also work when used to massage the reflex points on the bottom of your feet. You can also place the oil on your throat, chest, and back to get relief form coughing. The benefits of eucalyptus oil for coughs have even been recognized by commercial companies and is used in many products that people purchase for coughs. Many people do not realize that when you use eucalyptus oil you be able to more easily cough the mucus out of your chest. This is because the mucus will be loosened and easier to expel from your lungs.

289. Diabetes:

Diabetics will find that they can have increased circulation by using eucalyptus as described above. The best ways to receive the benefits is through massaging the oil on the body or to add it to your lotion. This should be done after a shower as that is the best time for improving circulation.

290. Disinfect:

You can use the antibacterial and antiviral properties of eucalyptus oil to naturally help to clean your home.

291. Dysentery:

Eucalyptus can be used to help treat dysentery when two drops are rubbed onto the stomach in a counter-clockwise direction. This will help to fight the infection, reduce inflammation and stop diarrhea.

292. Ear Aches:

While you should never put essential oils into the ear canal, they can be used to help with ear aches. Eucalyptus can help to reduce inflammation by massaging the oil around the outside of the ear. This should be done with just one drop to start and should be diluted in a carrier oil for children.

293. Emphysema:

You can use eucalyptus oil to really aid with respiratory disease. Diffusing eucalyptus oil and massaging one drop on the chest and one drop on the feet each day will help.

294. Expectorant:

You can use one drop of eucalyptus oil on the reflexology spots on the feet and one drop on the chest to help drain mucus from the lungs. This can be repeated up to three times each day as long as there is no issue with sensitivity to the oil.

295. Fever:

You can use eucalyptus oil to help reduce high fevers thanks to its cooling properties. It can really help to regulate the body temperature while aiding in the body's natural ability to fight infection.

296. Flu:

Eucalyptus uses when you have the flu will vary depending on the specific symptoms that you have. It can be used on the abdomen to help relieve stomach ailments, massaged onto achy muscles and joints, or just diffused throughout the home to help keep others from getting sick while helping to reduce the amount of time that you are sick.

297. Controlling Blood Sugar:

Massaging one or two drops of eucalyptus oil onto the soles of your feet each day will help you to regulate your blood sugar. Many researchers are currently trying to learn just how eucalyptus works to lower your lower blood sugar.

298. Inflammation:

When you have inflammation in an area you can massage one or two drops of eucalyptus oil onto the area in a motion that is towards your heart. This will help to support the lymphatic system in your body.

299. Iris Inflammation:

Eucalyptus oil can be used to help reduce the symptoms of iris inflammation. **The oil should never be put into the eye** but you can get the benefits by massaging it into your temples.

300. Jet Lag:

If you are suffering from jet lag, you can ease your symptoms by applying it topically or inhaling it.

301. Kidney Stones:

You can massage one or two drops of eucalyptus oil onto the affected kidney three times each day.

302. Lice:

You can treat lice naturally with eucalyptus oil because it is a natural insecticidal properties.

303. Measles:

You can diffuse eucalyptus oil into the home to reduce the length of the illness. You can also massage one or two drops of eucalyptus oil into the reflex points of your feet two or three times a day.

304. Neuralgia:

You can massage one or two drops of eucalyptus oil onto the affected areas to reduce the pain.

305. Neuritis:

You can massage drops of eucalyptus oil onto the reflex points on your feet and over the affected areas to reduce inflammation.

306. Overexercised Muscles:

Muscles that are overexercised often suffer from strain and fatigue and can be treated with a gentle massage using eucalyptus oil. You can massage the oil towards your heart to help move the lactic acid that cause the pain in the lymphatic system.

307. Pain:

When you are suffering from pain you should use eucalyptus oil by massaging it directly on the area of concern or the reflexology points associated with that area.

308. Pneumonia: To help clear your lungs you can diffuse eucalyptus oil and massaging it into your lungs and the reflexology points on your hands and feet.

309. Respiratory Viruses:

You can fight viral infections by using eucalyptus oil in a diffuser constantly when you are ill.

310. Rhinitis:

Inhaling eucalyptus oil from the bottle will help to open airways and reduce inflammation. It can also be massaged over the sinuses or added to a hot washcloth to be used as a hot compress.

311. Shingles:

Using eucalyptus oil for shingles will help with antiviral properties and easing inflation. It can be massaged onto the affected areas, added to a warm bath, or using a compress.

312. Sinusitis:

You can apply the eucalyptus oil to a hot washcloth to make a hot compress or you can add one or two drops to the reflex points of the feet. Eucalyptus oil can also be diffused into the room.

313. Tennis Elbow:

Massaging eucalyptus oil onto the area will help ease the pain of tennis elbow.

314. Tuberculosis:

You can use eucalyptus oil to fight bacterial infections, reduce inflammation, and clear the lungs. This can be done by diffusing until well and massaging two drops of eucalyptus oil onto the chest and back two or three times each day.

315. Pest Control:

You can also use eucalyptus oil to keep many dangerous pests and insects away. It is especially helpful with mosquitoes. Using eucalyptus oil mixed together with lemon oil will control pests well and is completely safe for pets and children.

316. Disinfectant:

Eucalyptus oil can be used to help fight infections in wounds. It will help to promote healing while fighting the inflammation that often hinders healing. This is a great option for someone who has minor burns or injuries.

317. Cold Sores:

You can sooth cold sores by using eucalyptus oil on them It will help with the healing process and will help to reduce pain.

318. Fresher Breath:

Eucalyptus oil can actually help to freshen your breath because of its antibacterial properties. This will help to combat the germs that are the cause of bad breath. While research is inconclusive on the subject many believe that eucalyptus oil can help to prevent plaque from building up on the teeth since it can work to treat the bacteria that attacks the gums and causes tooth decay.

319. Joint Pain:

You can ease join pain with eucalyptus oil. This is thanks to the oil's anti-inflammatory properties that help to ease pain.

Clove Oil Uses

For Health and Healing

Clove oil has a considerable number of benefits that can help with a variety of ailments. The following are some of the ways in which you can use clove oil. You can find cloves and clove oil easily but it is important if you are going to be ingesting the oil that you are choosing a therapeutic grade as some of the other grades of oils have additives that might not be safe for human consumption. Clove oil can also be dangerous so it is important to discuss your options and desired usage of clove oil with your health care provider before using it.

320. Addictions:

Clove oil can help you to reduce your desire for your addiction to tobacco. You can put a drop of clove oil on your tongue each time that you feel the need to smoke or chew tobacco. If the clove oil is a bit too strong for you, it can be diluted with coconut oil.

321. Antioxidant:

You can add clove oil to a veggie capsule or you can add it to your food to gain the benefits as a dietary supplement.

322. Athlete's Foot:

Clove oil can be used as a cure for athlete's foot by adding one or two drops to the area one or times each day.

323. Blood Clots:

To be able to help treat blood clots you can either add a few drops of clove oil to a veggie capsule and take as a supplement or you can massage one or two drops that have been diluted in a carrier oil over the area.

324. Boundaries:

To be able to help your heart you can massage clove oil over your heart or you diffuse.

325. Candida:

To treat candida you can use clove in a veggie capsule as a supplement that you take one a day for one or two weeks or you can dilute the oil with a carrier oil and massage onto a foot. Make sure that you alternate which foot you are massaging the oil onto each day. Ingesting clove oil can actually be a way to do a full candida cleanse of your digestive tract. This is something that can make you feel better and will help with your overall health. It will also boost your immune system when you do not have a candida problem which means that you are going to get sick less often.

326. Cataracts:

Cataracts are a bothersome condition of the eyes. While **clove oil should never be placed in the eye or in an area where it could get in the eye**, you can dilute one or two drops in a carrier oil and use to massage the reflex points on the feet and toes.

327. Codependency:

You can do a number of things that are going to help you with clove oil when you are struggling with codependency. You can inhale the oil from the bottle. You can also diffuse the oil while you are meditating or journalism. Clove oil can also be used topically as you are trying to figure out how you are going to work through a particular struggle.

328. Control Issues:

If you have problems with control and wanting to control things you can more easily learn how to let it go with the benefits of clove oil. To get these benefits diffuse clove oil throughout the day and then massage the oil into the feet.

329. Corns:

Diluting one drop of clove oil into several drops of a carrier oil like coconut oil and apply to the corn between one and three times each day will make it quickly go away.

330. Courage:

If you need courage for a situation you can gain it by diffusing clove oil into the room or inhaling it from the bottle.

331. Diarrhea:

For those suffering with diarrhea, you can calm your stomach naturally by massaging one or two drops of clove oil that have been diluted into coconut oil in a counter-clockwise direction on your stomach. This will really help to calm things down.

332. Digestive Issues:

People who have digestive issues can find relief when they take several drops of clove oil in a veggie capsule with food. They might also find that massaging the stomach with the clove oil can help with further problems.

333. Disinfectant:

You can disinfect your home with clove oil by diffusing into a room or making your own cleaning supplies and adding clove oil to them.

334. Empowerment:

When you need to feel empowered you can take matters into your own hands and gain more strength by inhaling clove oil or having it diffused throughout the room that you are in.

335. Fear:

If you live in fear of things like intimidation or rejection you can break these chains and start to feel better about yourself by diffusing the oil throughout your home. You can also inhale the oil directly from the bottle. You should think about doing this daily to boost your confidence and help you to keep these feelings under control.

336. Fever:

If you are suffering from a fever, you can add clove oil to a veggie capsule and take it internally. You can also use peppermint oil on the back of your neck at the same to help get quicker results.

337. Flatulence or Gas:

You can take clove oil internally as a dietary supplement and this is going to help you to reduce the amount of gas that you have in your stomach. In addition you can dilute the clove oil in a carrier oil like coconut oil and massage the lower stomach to help reduce the amount of gas build up that you have in your intestines.

338. Fungal Infections:

To get rid of a fungal infection you should mix one drop of clove oil with three drops of coconut oil and apply to the areas that are affected three times each day. You should do this until the infection has healed completely.

339. Heal Faster:

If you want to heal quickly then you only need to dilute clove oil in a carrier oil and massage that to the reflexology area that is associated with the area of concern.

340. Hepatitis Virus:

To help keep symptoms of the hepatitis virus controlled you can massage clove oil that has been diluted in a carrier oil onto one of your feet. You will want to switch the foot that you are using and alternate between them as you repeat daily.

341. Herpes Complex:

For the herpes complex you will want to dilute one drop of clove oil by mixing with three drops of coconut oil and then massaging onto alternate feet. You will want to use caution if you are working around your genitals as you clove oil is very strong and could burn.

342. Hodgkin's Disease:

For those suffering with Hodgkin's disease you can dilute the clove oil into a carrier oil and massage over the areas that you are concerned about one time each day.

343. Hormone:

To help balance hormones you can use one drop of clove oil that has been diluted and massage that onto the reflexology parts of your feet.

344. Hypothyroidism:

To help yourself with hypothyroidism you can apply one drop of the clove oil to your thyroid each day.

345. Infections:

You can apply one or two drops of diluted clove oil to the area of concern or on the reflexology points of the feet.

346. Insecticide:

There are a few ways that you can use clove oil as an insecticide. They include diffusing into a room or adding one drop of clove oil to a cotton ball and placing in the area of the home where the insects come into the house. You can also place these in places like behind the stove and fridge.

347. Intestinal Parasites:

To get rid of intestinal parasites you can take clove oil internally by putting several drops into a veggie capsule.

348. Liver Cleanse:

To cleanse your liver you can take clove oil internally. You will want to take several drops in a veggie capsule each day. You can also dilute clove oil and massage it into the liver or onto the reflexology points of the feet.

349. Lupus:

Those suffering from lupus will find relief when they take a few drops of clove oil in a veggie capsule with food. They can also find relief by massaging clove oil that has been diluted into a carrier oil onto the feet or any of the areas where they are feeling the effects of their condition.

350. Macular Degeneration:

To be able to manage macular generation, dilute clove oil into a carrier oil and massage on the reflex areas of the feet and toes each day. You can use a very diluted mixture of a carrier oil and clove oil on the temples but make sure that it is very diluted and be sure to avoid the eyes. You will also want to make sure to check your skin for sensitivity as this is a hot oil that has been known to burn some people.

351. Stimulate Memory:

To stimulate your memory when you are studying and working make sure that you diffuse clove oil into the area. You might also want to apply clove oil that has been diluted into a carrier oil to the back of your neck.

352. Balance Metabolism:

To help balance your metabolism you can diffuse clove oil. You can also inhale from the bottle or take internally by putting several drops into a veggie capsule and taking this with food.

353. Mold:

Clove oil can be used to get rid of mold and to kill the spores that cause it. You can diffuse clove oil throughout your home and you can also make a spray that contains clove oil that will get rid of the mold.

354. Muscle Pain and Muscle Aches:

When you have muscle pain and aches you can dilute the clove oil into a carrier oil and massage onto the areas that are sore.

355. Osteoporosis:

To be able to have relief from the symptoms of osteoporosis you can massage clove oil that has been diluted in a carrier roil to the areas that you are concerned about.

356. Poison Oak:

When you get poison oak you can dilute clove oil into a carrier oil and massage over the area. This is going to instantly remove the sting while helping to neutralize the poison making it go away faster.

357. Rheumatoid Arthritis:

Those suffering from rheumatoid arthritis are going to be able to find relief by massaging the joints with clove oil that has been diluted in a carrier oil one time each day. If they are experiencing pain at other times in the day this can be repeated. It is also going to help to provide an increase in circulation which can also benefit the person who is suffering from rheumatoid arthritis.

358. Ring Worm:

For someone suffering from ring worm, clove oil can be used to help get rid of the problem quickly. One or two time each day you can apply clove oil that has been diluted in a carrier oil directly the area where the ring worm is present.

359. Skin Cancer:

Someone who is suffering from skin cancer will find relief when they dilute clove oil in a carrier oil and apply to the area one or two times each day. This can help to keep the cancer from spreading. Other oils that can be used for this are sandalwood and frankincense.

360. Mouth Sores and Skin Sores:

If you have a sore in your mouth or on your skin then you can use clove oil to help the sore heal quickly. To do this you will want to dilute one drop of clove oil in a carrier oil and apply that to the sore one or two times each day until the sore has completely healed.

361. Thyroid Problems:

To help heal thyroid problems you can dilute one drop of clove oil into a carrier oil and rub over the thyroid each day.

362. Tooth Pain:

Dilute one drop of clove oil in one teaspoon of raw coconut oil and apply one or more drops to the desired area when you are suffering from tooth pain. Not only will this help the pain go away but it will also help to heal the problem that is causing the tooth pain. If you suffer from a dry socket then clove oil can be one of the best treatments for you. There are many different tooth issues that clove oil is beneficial in treating and reducing pain.

363. Teething:

To be able to get rid of teething pain, you can dilute one drop of clove oil into one tablespoon of raw coconut oil. Then you just apply this mixture as needed to the area that is bothering the child.

364. Lipoma Tumor:

For a lipoma tumor you can dilute one drop of clove oil into a carrier oil. You will then be able to apply this to the tumor or two times each day. It can help to reduce tumor size and keep the tumor from growing larger.

365. Leg Ulcer:

If you are suffering from a leg ulcer you can dilute clove oil into a carrier oil of choice and use that mixture to apply to the area of concern or to rub onto the reflexology point on the feet each day.

366. Viruses:

With viruses you can apply one or two drops of clove oil that has been diluted in a a carrier oil to the area where you are concerned about. You can also use the diluted oil on the reflex points of your feet between one and three times each day until you are well.

367. Warts:

When you have a wart that you would like to get rid of quickly take one drop of clove oil and dilute into three drops of coconut oil. Then apply this mixture to the wart one or two times each day until the wart is completely gone. Make sure that you have it completely gone or it will just come back over time.

368. Wounds:

If you have a wound and you would like to use the benefits of clove oil to keep it from being infected and to help it heal quickly then you just need to dilute your clove oil and then apply to the area of concern. If this is too painful then you can also apply the mixture to your feet in the area for reflexology.

369. Moisturize Skin:

Many people do not realize that clove oil is great for moisturizing dry skin and curing many additional skin problems that you might have. If you want to use clove oil as a remedy for dry skin then you need to get the oil in liquid form. You will want to put the oil on a clean rag and then spread it on your skin. You might need to dilute the clove oil in a carrier oil.

370. Skin Irritation:

If you have an area that is irritated in some way then you can use clove oil to help sooth the area. It works great to help sooth itching and burning when it is diluted in a carrier oil.

371. Increase Your Libido:

Those who are having a hard time with their sexual energy levels can add one drop of clove oil to their coffee or any other beverage. It can quickly help to increase your sex drive.

372. Stomach Pain:

If you suffer from stomach pain you can use clove oil to help you. Clove has actually been years for hundreds of years for stomach pain and illnesses that had to do with the stomach. You can add a few drops of clove to your beverage to get these stomach settling benefits.

373. Antioxidant:

Clove oil also has a lot of antioxidant power. It can contain more than thirty times the amount of anti-oxidants that are in blueberries. Antioxidants reduce the damage of free radicals which can cause cancer and cell death. Antioxidants also slow the aging process, slow degeneration, and help to protect the body against viruses and bacteria. Since clove oil has such strong protective qualities it is often used in oil blends that are known for protection and healing.

IN YOUR HOUSE:

374. Termites:

If you want to keep termites away you can diffuse clove oil in the house or you can add it to cotton balls that you place around your home.

375. Clean Metals:

Not only is clove oil good for you it can also be helpful for many things that you might have laying around your home. You can soak a clean cotton rag in clove oil and use that to clean many metal surfaces that might need to be cleaned.

376. Weed Killer:

Many people hate weeds but hate the harmful chemicals that are in weed killers. One great thing about clove oil is that it is one of the best weed killers that you can find. Using clove oil as a weed killer is also safe which makes it a great option for home gardens. Plus it will keep the pests away too.

377. Cooking Odors:

Have you ever cooked something that left a lingering odor in your home that was less than pleasant. Putting clove oil on a cotton ball in the room, diffusing the oil, or making a spray can help you to reduce the times that you notice these oils. Plus if you do notice them you can quickly make them go away.

CINNAMON OIL USES

Cinnamon oil has a lot of great things that it can do for your body and the air that you breathe. Cinnamon is an essential oil that everyone will want to have in their home when they realize all of the great benefits that it has.

FOR HEALTH AND HEALING

378. Airborne Bacteria:

Cinnamon oil is great for diffusing during winter months, cold, and flu season. It is also great to diffuse when someone in your house is sick and you do not want everyone else to be ill. Adding cinnamon oil to a cotton ball and sticking in your car's vent while you drive is another way to help kill all of the airborne bacteria that you might come into contact with.

379. Bacterial Infections:

There are many things that you can do if you want to help cure bacterial infections with cinnamon oil. You can diffuse the oil and even apply it topically. If you are applying topically the recommendation is to dilute the oil into a carrier oil. You can then massage over the area where there is an infection.

380. Bites or Stings:

When you have a bug bite or a sting you can use one drop of cinnamon oil with three drops of carrier oil and apply it to the area. This is going to help with the irritation as well as helping to prevent an infection.

381. Breathing Issues:

If you suffer from respiratory issues like asthma then you should diffuse cinnamon oil into the area. You can also dilute the cinnamon oil and massage it on the neck and chest.

382. Diabetes:

Cinnamon oil is a great choice for diabetics because it has been shown to help regulate blood sugar. You can add cinnamon oil to your food or take one or two drops in a veggie capsule. It is also possible to use the oil (diluted into a carrier oil) to rub over your pancreas.

383. Diverticulitis:

If you want to help heal diverticulitis then you can use cinnamon oil that has been diluted to massage your stomach. This not only promotes healing but will also help to decrease inflammation.

384. Fungal Infections:

Anyone who is worried about a fungal infection should start diffusing cinnamon oil into the air. Then they should dilute the cinnamon oil into a carrier oil to massage onto the area of concern or to rub into the soles of the feet for fast absorption.

385. Improve Moods:

If you need to find something uplifting to improve your moods you can diffuse the cinnamon oil into the air. You can also add a few drops to your bath water or use it topically but diluting it first is recommended.

386. Immune System Booster:

During cold and flu season you can help to make sure that you stay well by diffusing cinnamon oil. It is also great to make a steam tent by boiling water over the stove and adding a few drops of cinnamon oil. Then you just hold your head over the pot while draping a towel around you. (Do not do this while a burner is on for safety reasons. It is also recommended that you remove the pan from the burner before making the tent.)

387. Infection Control:

If you have an infection one of the best ways to quickly and naturally cure the infection is to massage diluted cinnamon oil onto the soles of the feet. You can also diffuse the oil throughout the area that you are in.

388. Stimulate Your Libido:

Using cinnamon oil topically on the lower abdomen is a great way to help improve your sex drive. You will want to make sure that you do not get the oil near your genitals though. You can also use the oil aromatically to help improve your libido.

389. Support the Pancreas:

Cinnamon oil is known to help promote healthy pancreas function. Massaging cinnamon oil that has been diluted in a carrier oil to the pancreas or to the soles of the feet can help. You can also add the cinnamon oil to your cooking and take internally for these benefits.

390. Battle Fatigue:

Cinnamon oil can help increase circulation, improve energy levels, and increase blood flow to the brain when you are able to use it aromatically. You can add it to your bath, inhale it from the bottle, or diffuse it for these benefits.

391. Fight Pneumonia:

If someone has pneumonia they can diffuse cinnamon oil throughout the home to aid and speed up the healing process.

392. Typhoid:

Typhoid is a bacteria infection that you could get rid of with the use of cinnamon oil. You should dilute the cinnamon oil into a carrier oil and have it used for a full body massage or used on the soles of your feet. It is also a good idea to have it diffused throughout the home.

393. Vaginitis:

If you have a vaginitis or a vaginal infection then diluted cinnamon oil can help you with fighting the infections. You will want to make sure that you are cautious and check for sensitivity. Avoid contact with the genitals and massage into your lower stomach.

394. Viruses:

You can also use cinnamon oil to help you with viral infections. The best way to get the benefits for this is to use the cinnamon oil and dilute it in a carrier oil. Then you can massage it into the area of concern, over the soles of you feet, or your entire body.

395. Warming:

Cinnamon oil does the opposite of what peppermint oil does and it helps to warm you. This is a great thing to use in the winter when you can massage diluted cinnamon oil over your heart, around your neck, or on the soles of the feet to help you feel warm when you are cold.

There are some additional things that cinnamon oil can be good for that you might want to take note of. Cinnamon oil can help to boost circulation, fight coughs, fight colds, aid in digestion, reduce inflammation, remove warts, and increase energy.

IN YOUR HOUSE

396. Fight Mold, Fungus, and Mildew:

If you have issues with mold, fungus, or mildew you can fight it by using cinnamon oil in the area. You can add cinnamon oil to your favorite cleaners or make your own natural cleaner with the oil. You can also diffuse it regularly to areas where it is more prone to mold and mildew.

FOR USE WITH FOOD

397. Cooking:

Cinnamon oil is a great addition to your kitchen as well. You can easily apply the oil to your favorite recipes to add that cinnamon flavor that you desire. Do keep in mind that you want to be using therapeutic grade oils if you are going to be using them in foods.

CASSIA OIL USES

FOR HEALTH AND HEALING

398. Antiseptic:

Using cassia oil as an antiseptic is a very common use. You need to dilute the cassia oil in a carrier oil and then apply it to the reflexology points on your feet.

399. Colds:

If you have a cold you might want to diffuse cassia oil throughout your home. You can add one or two drops of cassia oil to a veggie capsule to take internally.

400. Digestion Issues:

If you have issues with your digestive system you can dilute the cassia oil with a carrier oil to be massaged into the soles of your feet at the reflex points. You can also massage onto your stomach or take one drop internally.

401. Flu:

If you have the flu or have been exposed to the flu then you can try to combat it by diffusing cassia oil throughout your home and taking internally by adding one or two drops of cassia oil to veggie capsules.

402. Fungal Infection:

If you are suffering from a fungal infection you will want to apply a small about of the cassia oil that has been diluted with a carrier oil directly to the area of concern one or two times each day.

403. H Pylori:

If you have H Pylori you will want to take cassia oil internally in a veggie capsule or on food. You also can dilute the oil in a carrier oil to be massaged on the stomach.

404. Support Immune System Health:

Diffusing cassia oil in your home can help to boost your immune system naturally. You can also massage one drop of the cassia oil that has been diluted into a carrier oil onto your feet.

405. Reduce Digestive Inflammation:

If you are worried about inflammation in your digestive system then you can take cassia oil internally in a veggie capsule or in food. You can also massage the stomach with cassia oil that has been diluted in a carrier oil.

406. Ringworm:

If you see ringworm you can get rid of it by diluting cassia oil in a carrier oil and then applying to the area one or two times each day.

407. Viral Infections:

If you are worried about a viral infection you can apply cassia oil that has been diluted to the area one or two times each day. You can also take internally from a veggie capsule.

408. Cure Diarrhea:

Cassia can really work wonders on helping to cure and heal ailments of the digestive tract. Cassia oil can actually be used as something to help stop diarrhea. It can bind the bowels to stop episodes while curing through its microbial properties. This actually stops the diarrhea from occurring and helps to bind the stool with fiber.

409. Antidepressant:

You can fight depression with cassia oil since it can induce warm feelings in both the mind and body and help to uplift moods.

410. Anti-emetic:

If you feel nauseous or are vomiting you can use cassia oil to stop it. This is because cassia oil actually helps to induce a refreshing feeling that will keep the feelings of being sick away.

411. Anti-galactogogue:

Cassia oil should not be handled or used by lactating mothers as it can reduce the secretion of milk.

412. Helps with Arthritis and Rheumatoid Arthritis:

Cassia oil helps to stimulate the circulatory system. It is going to improve the blood circulation while helping to make the joints and other parts of the body that are affected warm. This can be taken internally via a veggie capsule or you can use it to massage and treat the areas that are sore but it is generally recommended that you dilute it in a carrier oil first.

413. Antimicrobial:

Cassia oil will inhibit the growth of microbial and protect from microbial infections. This can be used in a variety of body parts like the colon, urethra, kidneys, and urinary tract to name a few.

414. Improved Circulation:

Cassia oil actually helps to improve the circulation of the blood which can help to take oxygen and nutrients to the different parts of the body. This is one of the ways in which cassia oil can help with things like arthritis and rheumatoid arthritis.

415. Antiviral:

You can counter viral infections and help protect your body from a cold, influenza, cough, and may other viral infections by using cassia oil on a regular basis. Diffusing cassia oil throughout your home is the best way to get these powerful benefits.

416. Reduce Cramping:

Cassia oil can also be used to help relax the muscles that cause menstrual cramps. The oil will help to open up the obstructed menstruation paths. It will also help with addition symptoms of PMS like drowsiness, nausea, and headaches.

417. Fever:

Since cassia oil works as both an antiviral and antimicrobial agent it is great at fighting infections that cause fevers. It can also help to lower the body's temperature. Plus with the circulatory properties it is able to really boost the immune system throughout the body. Even thought the oil has a warming effect it is still able to help reduce fevers.

418. Stimulant:

Cassia oil is a great essential oil to take internally on a regular basis. It will help to stimulate many different functions from within the body. It helps with secretions, circulation, the nervous system, functions of the brain, discharges, and metabolism and can help you to be more alert and active when you inhale it or are in a room where it is being diffused.

419. Gas Relief:

Cassia oil will offer relief in the intestines from gasses and will help to force them out of the body. Plus it will help to keep future gases from forming.

420. Hemorrhaging:

Finally thanks to the astringent properties of cassia oil, it can be used to help alleviate many different types of hemorrhaging.

IN YOUR HOME

421. Repel Insects:

Diffusing cassia oil in a room is a natural way to keep insects away. You can create a spray using five drops of cassia oil to every ounce of water or you can add a cotton ball that has cassia oil on it to a place where insects are likely to be.

FOR USE WITH FOOD

422. Cooking:

Cassia oil can be used as a flavoring agent when cooking. Make sure that you start slow and add one drop at a time.

CARDAMOM OIL USES

Cardamom has a number of beneficial uses. There are so many things that you can use cardamom for that you might even find yourself diffusing this helpful oil all of the time. Here are some of the uses for cardamom.

FOR HEALTH AND HEALING

423. Anger:

If you are feeling angry you can reduce the feelings of anger by diffusing cardamom oil in the room that you are in.

424. Increase in Appetite:

You can help to increase your appetite if you inhale cardamom from the bottle or massage one or two drops onto the stomach. This is great for people who have illnesses that make them not want to eat.

425. Asthma:

For asthma you can massage cardamom oil over your chest and inhale from your hands. You can also diffuse. Cardamom can also reduce symptoms of asthma when you massage the reflex points with one or two drops of the oil. You can also place a small drop of the oil underneath the nose.

426. Bacterial Infections:

To rid yourself of bacterial infections you can use cardamom oil topically. You can put the oil on the area multiple times throughout the day.

427. Blame:

If you are battling with feelings of blame you can diffuse multiple drops of cardamom oil throughout the room. This will help to instantly improve your moods.

428. Bronchitis:

To be able to get rid of bronchitis put a few drops of cardamom oil in hot water to make a steam tent and breathe deeply. Do not heat the water to a boiling point.

429. Congestion:

If you are congested you can prepare a steam tent as described above. You can also use a diffuser or massage one or two drops of the cardamom oil to the area of concern.

430. Cough:

If you have a cough you can massage one or two drops of cardamom oil on the reflex points on your feet or on the chest.

431. Diarrhea:

If you have diarrhea then you can massage one or two drops of the cardamom oil in a counter-clockwise direction on the abdomen. You can do this every fifteen minutes. With cardamom oil it is better to use less oil with a more frequent application for the treatment of diarrhea.

432. Digestive System:

If you are struggling with digestion issues you can apply one or two drops of cardamom topically. You can also take it internally in a veggie capsule or on food or inhale directly from the bottle.

433. Edema:

When you are suffering from edema you can massage one or two drops of cardamom oil gently in the area that you are concerned about. Make sure that you are massaging in a direction that is towards the heart.

434. Balance Emotions:

If you are struggling with your emotions you can diffuse cardamom oil throughout your room or home. You can also massage the cardamom oil over the different energy centers in the body.

435. Gas:

For someone who is suffering with gas you can add one drop of cardamom oil to a glass of water or you can add between one and three drops of cardamom oil to a veggie capsule to take internally. You can also massage over the lower part of your stomach.

436. Food Poisoning:

There are several things that you can do with cardamom oil if you are suffering from food poisoning. You can add between one and three drops of cardamom oil to a glass of water. You can massage the oil onto the stomach or the reflex points n your feet. Finally you can inhale the oil from your hands or directly from the bottle.

437. Feeling Frustrated:

If you are feeling frustrated you can diffuse cardamom oil throughout the room.

438. Halitosis:

Halitosis can be treated by placing a small amount of cardamom oil on the tongue. You can all use one drop internally each day to really help cure problems from chronic bad breath.

439. Headache

:To be able to get rid of headaches you can inhale deeply after putting one drop of cardamom oil on your palms. You can also massage the oil directly into the areas where you feel tension.

440. Indigestion:

You can use between one and two drops of cardamom oil internally each day to get rid of indigestion. You can also apply topically and smell the oil as often as every twenty to thirty minutes when you are struggling with indigestion. With cardamom oil it is better to use the oil more often in smaller amounts to get the maximum benefits.

441. Infections:

If you have an infection you can use the oil to help treat the infected area. Starting off with just one drop you can move up from there when you determine how much you need. It is better to increase the frequency as opposed to increasing the amount of the oil that you are using each application.

442. Inflammation:

For inflammation you can massage the cardamom oil over the area of concern or you can try a drop of cardamom oil in a glass of water or veggie capsule for inflammation in the digestive tract.

443. Invigorate:

If you are hoping to be able to cash in on the invigorating properties of cardamom oil you can inhale a drop from your hands or add it to food for a boost of flavor.

444. Achy Muscles:

Those suffering with achy muscles will find that they can get relief with a massage using one or two drops of the oil over the entire area. You can also get a full body massage using the oil.

445. Spasms in the Muscles:

Massaging one or two drops of cardamom oil into the area where you are experiencing a muscle spasm can help to relieve the problem.

446. Nausea:

If you are experiencing nausea you can inhale cardamom oil from your hands, massage a drop of the oil onto your stomach, or even put a drop on your tongue.

447. Respiratory Issues:

People suffering from respiratory issues will find a number of benefits and relief when they use a drop under their nose, massage one or two drops on the chest, or diffuse into the area where they are at.

448. Be More Responsible:

To be more responsible you can diffuse cardamom oil into the room where you are at. You can also inhale from your hands.

449. Spasms in the Stomach:

For someone who is suffering from stomach spasms they can find relief when they massage their stomach with cardamom oil, take one or two drops internally through a veggie capsule, or by drinking one or two drops in water.

450. Ulcers:

If you have an ulcer you can regularly add cardamom oil to the food that you are eating. You can also take one drop internally each day.

451. Mood Benefits:

Cardamom oil has uplifting benefits that can improve your mood. You can get these benefits by massaging one or two drops over the chest or diffusing in the room that you are in.

452. Vomiting:

If you have been sick and vomiting a drop of cardamom oil on the tongue or massaged on the stomach can help. You can also diffuse the cardamom oil in the room.

453. Maintains Health:

Cardamom oil has a number of vitamins that help to maintain your health and boost your immune system. Some of the vitamins that are found in cardamom oil are Vitamin C, Vitamin B3, and Vitamin B2. The oil also has a number of the minerals that are essential for health including iron, manganese, magnesium, calcium, potassium, and copper. Cardamom oil also has antioxidant properties.

454. Boost Health:

If you want to boost your health then taking cardamom oil is going to really help. This is because there are so many minerals and vitamins that it is going to help to metabolite cellular energy as well as help with generating red blood cells. In addition it can help to improve cardiovascular health and provide antioxidant properties.

455. Kidneys:

Cardamom oil is a natural diuretic that can help to make urine discharge from your body. This can help to keep kidneys free from calcium deposited, urea, and other toxins. It also will help to reduce blood pressure and help with weight loss.

456. Body Temperature:

Cardamom oil is also known to maintain body temperature. It can help us to heat up to have the normal body temperature. It can even help us to sweat to maintain that body temperature. Plus it will help with relieving headaches and curing common ailments like the cold and a cough.

FOR BEAUTY

457. Skin Benefits:

There are a number of benefits that you can gain from using cardamom oil on the skin. It can help to give skin a healthy glow and disinfect. It can be used as a natural cleanser and/or toner.

458. Hair Benefits:

Cardamom oil also offers a number of benefits to your hair. You can help to treat infections on your scalp, maintain your hair's health, cure dandruff, and even lighten hair naturally.

FOR USE WITH FOOD

459. Cooking:

If you are cooking with the cardamom oil then you will want to start using very little. A little bit of cardamom oil goes a very long way.

GRAPEFRUIT OIL USES

Grapefruit oil must be purchased at a therapeutic or medical grade in order to get these benefits. This does not apply to all essential oil brands. Sadly industry standards do not regulate natural or pure products so many essential oils on the market are not therapeutic grade and can end up making you sick. Make sure that you choose an essential oil that is therapeutic grade especially if you are going to be ingesting it and taking it internally. Here are some of the many benefits of using grapefruit oil.

Beware: There can be some interactions with some medicine, talk to your physician first.

FOR HEALTH AND HEALING

460. Curb Your Addictions:

People who suffer from food and even drug cravings will find that the grapefruit aroma uplifts their spirit and their system. To get these benefits you can apply one or two drops of the oil over the stomach or the back of the neck. You can also just inhale from the bottle or diffuse.

461. Anorexia:

People suffering from anorexia can gain benefits from grapefruit oil as it helps to uplift their moods and helps them to have a higher sense of self. It can also increase an appetite that has been depressed when used aromatically by inhaling from a bottle or diffusing into a room.

462. Suppression of Appetite:

While the grapefruit oil will help increase appetite in someone with a depressed appetite it will work the opposite way with people who are having food cravings or are stuck in the rut of emotional eating. It can even help you to reduce binge eating when you are inhaling the scent on a regular basis.

463. Bulimia:

Since grapefruit oil improves ones sense of self it will also help to uplift the mood and increase the depressed appetite when inhaled.

464. Cardiovascular System Help:

To get the support of cardiovascular support you just need to add a drop of grapefruit oil to your lotion and massage each night towards your heart.

465. Cellulite:

You can help to reduce cellulite by mixing one or two drops of grapefruit oil with coconut oil and massaging into the body in a kneading pattern each evening.

466. Digestion:

Help to stimulate your digestive system by adding a drop of grapefruit oil to your water or massaging the oil into your abdomen.

467. Cure a Dry Throat:

You can cure a dry throat by adding one or two drops of grapefruit oil to a cup of warm water. You will gargle first and then swallow. You can do this as often as needed. You can also add a drop of grapefruit oil to a teaspoon of coconut oil and then swish it through your mouth gargling. You can swallow this or you can spit it out.

468. Improve Fatigue:

If you want to be able to naturally cure your fatigue you can increase your energy levels by diffusing grapefruit oil or you can apply a drop of the oil to your chest.

469. Edema:

Mixing one or two drops of grapefruit oil with coconut oil and massing over the area in a direction that is towards the heart three or four times each day will help to cure edema. You can also help the body's expulsion process by putting several drops of the oil in your water.

470. Gallbladder Stones:

To help cure gallbladder stones you can massage one or two drops of grapefruit oil over the area or onto the soles of your feet. You can also mix with peppermint oil in support of a healthy digestive system.

471. Cure a Hangover:

To get rid of a hangover quick you can diffuse or inhale grapefruit oil directly from the bottle. It really does have an effect that is quite surprising with your hangovers. You can also add one or two drops to each glass of water that you are drinking. It is important when you are hung over to drink two or three times the normal amount of water that you usually drink for two or three days to rehydrate your body.

472. Help with Jet Lag:

Using grapefruit oil to help increase your energy levels by inhaling or adding it to your water bottles will help prevent jet lag.

473. Support Your Kidneys:

To help with kidney issues you can massage grapefruit oil over your lower back and stomach. You can also add it to smoothies or water.

474. Help Your Liver:

You can help to cleanse your body of unwanted toxins by adding grapefruit oil to your smoothies and water. You can also massage the grapefruit oil on your liver.

475. Lymphatic Help:

You can help to cleanse your lymphatic system and to decongestant lymph nodes as well. The best way to do this is to add a drop of the grapefruit oil to your lotion and to massage the lotion onto your skin. You will want to massage starting at your hands and feet in a direction towards your heart.

476. Reduce Stress:

One of the best ways to reduce the mental stress that you feel is to rub grapefruit oil through your hair to diffuse into the room. You will be creating mental clarity and helping to uplift your mind while increasing your confidence. You can also use grapefruit oil topically in a lotion, in your bath, or put a drop on your heart.

477. Relieve Migraines:

If you have a migraine headache you can find relief when you are reducing stress by applying the oil topically or using in an aromatic way.

478. After a Miscarriage:

If you have had a miscarriage you can improve your emotional and physical healing by massaging grapefruit oil into the body and onto the soles of your feet.

479. Fight Obesity:

Using grapefruit oil aromatically throughout the day will help to decrease your appetite and help you to lose weight. You can also use it topically throughout the day when you start to feel stress. Plus you can a few drops to your water so that you will drink more water and get flavor in a natural healthy way.

480. Don't Overeat:

You can also decrease your binge eating and reduce cravings by diffusing the oil or inhaling it directly from the bottle. Using grapefruit oil as a perfume can also help you to not struggle with overeating as much.

481. Stress Over Performance:

If you are constantly stressed by how you will perform in certain situations then you need grapefruit oil. You can add the oil to your bath, add it to your water that you are drinking, massage the solar plexus with it, or just diffuse it into the room that you are in so that you can increase yourself of self and balance.

482. PMS:

If you are suffering from PMS you should put grapefruit oil on your wrist or shirt collar as a perfume. You can also add it to your bath or massage it over your stomach and soles of your feet. This is going to help balance and regulate hormones.

483. Decrease risk of Skin Cancer:

If you simply add grapefruit oil to your water and massage it in the skin each evening you can decrease skin cancer. It is important to massage into areas where you have had higher rates of sun exposure but make sure that you avoid direct sunlight after you have put the oil on as it will make you more sensitive to the sun.

484. Stop Craving Sugar:

Inhaling grapefruit oil when you have a sugar craving will help you to reduce caving into that craving. You can also add the grapefruit oil to your water between one and three times each day to take it as a supplement.

485. Withdrawal:

You can stop having symptoms of withdrawal by diffusing grapefruit oil or rubbing it onto your neck and throat.

486. Disinfect:

Since grapefruit oil has natural antimicrobial and antiviral properties it is a great disinfectant. It can protect the body from getting new infections while helping to eliminate any infections that are currently present. It can also help to treat infections that are in the stomach, colon, urinary system, intestines, kines, and excretory system. It can also help to heal infections that are on the skin.

487. Antiseptic:

You can also use the antiseptic properties of grapefruit oil to benefit you when you apply the oil to acne, cuts, wounds, or bruises. This will help to protect from infections that are microbial as well as preventing you from developing tetanus or becoming septic.

488. Stimulate:

There are many ways in which grapefruit oil will stimulate the body. The oil will help your brain by making it more active while helping to give your thoughts new direction. It will also stimulate the endocrine glands and support hormone secretion. Your body can improve its metabolism and keep it in order with the help of grapefruit oil. You can also help to stimulate the nervous system and become more alert and active. Grapefruit oil also helps to stimulate the secretion of bile and gastric juices in the stomach which will help to move food that has not been digested through the intestines. It can even help to simulate the circulatory system, excretory system, and lymphatic system.

489. Depression:

You can help to treat depression with grapefruit oil as it will help with making you have feelings of hope and relieving stress or anxiety.

490. Dry Mouth:

Mixing together one or two drops of grapefruit oil in warm water and gargling will help to relieve a dry mouth. You can add a drop of oil to one teaspoon of coconut oil as well. You can swallow both of these when you are done gargling.

FOR BEAUTY

491. Hair:

Grapefruit oil can really help the hair to maintain its natural sheen and shine.

GRAPE SEED OIL USES

Beware: There can be some interactions with some medicine, talk to your physician first.

Grape seed oil has been known for its many benefits to the skin. You will be able to use grape seed in a number of ways and it also works great as a carrier oil for essential oils.

FOR HEALTH AND HEALING

492. Antioxidants:

Grapeseed oil contains the flavonoid oligomeric procyanidin which is one of the strongest antioxidants. It can help to fight against cell damage and tissue damage that can occur because of free radicals.

493. Heart:

Your hear will be healthier when you take grape seed oil internally because it helps to lower the bad cholesterol while boosting the level of good cholesterol. It reduces your risk for heart disease and keeps your heart healthy.

494. Diabetes:

Diabetics will benefit from grape seed oil because it has linoleic acid which has been proven to be beneficial in controlling blood sugar.

495. Blood Vessels and Capillaries:

Grape seed oil will help to repair broken and damaged blood vessels and capillaries. It will help to sooth problems like varicose veins and spider veins while helping to improve circulation of the blood.

496. Inflammation:

If you have pain from inflammation and swelling from arthritis then you can use grape seed oil to treat the symptoms.

497. Prevent Cancer:

Recent studies have shown that grape seed oil can help to prevent many different types of cancer including prostate cancer, lung cancer, breast cancer, stomach cancer, and prostate cancer. You can get the antioxidant benefits by using at least one tablespoon of grapeseed oil in your food daily. This will help to prevent these types of cancer and more.

498. After Surgery:

After you have had sugar you can use grape seed oil for some amazing benefits. It will help to reduce the swelling faster which will promote healing.

499. Wounds:

You can help wounds to heal quickly by using grape seed oil on them.

500. Sealant:

Grape seed oil can be used to seal in moisture in your skin and hair.

501. Enhance Moisture:

If you have a current moisturizer that you like but do not feel like it helps to moisturize your skin enough then you can enhance that moisturizer with grape seed oil.

502. With Whipped Butter:

You can mix grapeseed oil into whipped butter to help you have more healthy butter and to be able to get the grapeseed oil that you need in your diet.

503. Hot Oil Treatment:

You can also use grape seed oil to do you own hot oil treatment for your hair prior to washing.

FOR BEAUTY

ON YOUR FACE

To use grapeseed oil on your face you will want to put a few drops of the oil onto your hands and massage in an upward direction. It will quickly be absorbed into your skin.

504. Relieve Acne:

If you have problems with acne you can use grape seed oil to improve the quality of your skin. You can reduce a number of skin problems with regular use. This includes that it can help to prevent pores from clogging. You can prevent acne outbreaks and help to cure existing outbreaks.

505. Tighten the Skin:

You can also use grape seed oil to tone and tighten the skin. It is a very good choice for people who have oily skin.

506. Under-Eye Circles:

If you have dark circles under your eyes it can make your skill look lifeless and dull. Grape seed oil can easily help you to reduce under-eye circles naturally without being dangerous.

507. Moisturize Your Skin:

If you need moisture you can use grape seed oil to cure it. This will leave your skin soft and smooth without making it feel greasy.

508. Prevent Aging in the Skin:

If you have fine lines and wrinkles then you should use grape seed oil to keep you from looking older. Using grape seed oil regularly will help to reduce the aging process.

ON YOUR HAIR

509. Hair Growth:

You can use grape seed oil on your hair to help nourish the hair and scalp which will help your hair to grow faster.

510. Moisturize Your Hair and Scalp:

You can use grape seed oil to keep your hair feeling soft and moisturized and to help keep hair thick, repair split ends, and avoid breaking.

511. Dandruff:

You can get rid of dandruff with grape seed oil.

512. Add Shine to Hair:

When you use grape seed oil on your hair it is going to shine more.

513. Strengthen Hair:

You are also going to help to strengthen you hair with the use of grape seed oil.

514. Condition:

Grape seed oil is a natural conditioner for hair and it works great with dry and brittle hair. It can even help you to have the hair that you need to get the latest trendy style that you want.

515. No Allergens:

Grape seed oil does not contain any allergens so it can work on even the most sensitive scalp.

Frankincense Oil Uses

For Health and Healing

516. Uterine Health:

You can help promote uterine health with frankincense oil as it helps to control the production of estrogen. It will also prevent cysts from forming in the uterus as well as preventing tumors after menopause (this is the leading cause of uterine cancer). Frankincense oil will also help you to have regular menstruation and with many other gynecologic conditions.

517. Astringent:

Frankincense is also an astringent that is known for strengthening in the hair roots by contracting the blood vessels. It helps to strengthen gums, strengthen the intestine and internal muscles, and can prevent premature hair loss. You can also get relief from diarrhea with the oil and help to keep those ab muscles firm. You can even use frankincense to help slow bleeding in wounds or cuts.

518. Asthma:

Frankincense oil is one of the best home remedies for asthma and you can gain the benefits by breathing from the bottle, diffusing it into the air, or rubbing the oil on your palms. You can also rub the oil on your feet and toes or apply to the chest and spine.

519. Oral Health:

You can improve your oral health with frankincense oil reducing mouth sores, toothaches, bad breath and mouth infections.

520. Mental Health:

You can improve your mental health and mental clarity with frankincense oil. You can apply this at the back of your neck of inhale from the bottle.

521. Digestion:

Frankincense is known to improve severe indigestion and acidity because it treats the digestion process and does more than just overpower it like many of the popular medications available on the market today. It fastens the secretion of gastric juices that are in the stomach to keep the food moving quickly and easily through the intestines.

522. Fight Cancer Cells:

Many studies have proven that you can fight cancer cells with frankincense oil. In fact frankincense oil has been proven to kill bladder cancer cells in studies.

523. Radiant Skin:

Keep your skin looking radiant and healthy with frankincense oil. The oil will help to regenerate kin cells which means that t can help with scars, skin pocks, cuts, and stretch marks. It even helps to rid the body of precancerous and cancerous moles. Using frankincense oil with coconut oil each day will keep the skin looking radiant and healthy.

524. Hormonal Balance:

You can use frankincense oil to help regulate the pituitary gland and the hypothalamus. The hypothalamus is the main glad that produces growth hormones and controls the thyroid.

525. Depression:

Frankincense oil will hep to treat depression because it helps to stimulate the limbic system that is present in the brain.

526. Immune Support:

You can use frankincense oil to help improve your immune system. You just need to apply between one and three drops to the bottoms of your feet to get this boost in your immune system. It will also help you to quickly get rid of coughs and colds.

527. Alzheimer's Disease:

You can help someone with Alzheimer's disease to have mental clarity by diffusing frankincense oil into their room or by adding to their shirt color or pillow. It can also be used for a full body massage or to massage the feet.

528. Aneurysm:

To help with an aneurysm you can inhale frankincense through a steam team or massage onto the reflex points on your feet.

529. Arthritis:

Frankincense can be used in the treatment of arthritis by inhaling daily through steam and massing into the joints.

530. Balance:

Frankincense oil can help you to feel overwhelmed by diffusing into the room and massaging into your feet.

531. Brain:

You can help prevent aging in the brain by inhaling the frankincense oil and apply it topically or massaging it into your body or feet. It can also be used in your bath or can be diffused. This also works to restore mental clarity after a brain injury.

532. Breathing:

See asthma above.

533. Coma:

If someone is in a coma you can use frankincense oil to help keep the muscles from getting atrophy by massaging into the hands and feet as well as all over the entire body.

534. Concussion:

You can add a drop of frankincense oil to steaming water and inhale in a steam tent. You can also use the oil to massage into the toes and feet if you have a concussion.

535. Confused:

If you are confused you can add frankincense oil behind your ears, on your shirt collar, or diffuse through the home.

536. Fibroid:

When suffering from fibroid you can massage the frankincense oil into the reflexology points on the feet, use several drops in a bath, or apply the oil to a hot compress.

537. Genital Warts:

You can get rid of genital warts by dabbing the oil on the wart each day once a day until it is gone.

538. Hepatitis:

Hepatitis can be cured through inhaling frankincense oil in a steam tent and massaging two drops into each of the hands and feet every day.

539. Vision:

You can see clearly and improve your vision when you massage frankincense oil into your toes and the tips of your fingers.

540. Wound Infections:

You can help to heal wounds that are infected quickly with frankincense oil. You will be able to do this by inhaling it through a steam tent, adding a drop to warm water and soaking the should, or creating a spray that contains distilled water and several drops of frankincense oil. You can also diffuse frankincense oil throughout the house.

541. Cirrhosis of the Liver:

You can get improvement from cirrhosis by massaging the frankincense oil over the liver and the outside of your right foot. You can also inhale directly from the bottle.

542. Lou Gehrig's Disease:

Lou Gehrig's Disease can be treated by inhaling one or two drops of frankincense oil through a steam tent. You can also massage the entire body moving in a direction towards the heart and massage the soles of the feet each day.

543. Prayer and Meditation:

Using frankincense oil in a diffuser during your times of prayer and medication will help to make you feel more connected. You can also rub on the hands, feet, or over your head.

544. Memory:

You can improve mental clarity and memory by adding one or two drops of frankincense oil to a steam tent or diffusing while you are studying or trying to memorize something.

545. Fatigue:

When you are feeling mentally fatigued you can add frankincense to your bath water or massage the oil into your scalp and across your chest.

546. After a Miscarriage:

When you have a miscarriage you can seek relief from frankincense oil. You will want to massage the oil on the abdomen, around the ankle, and over the feet. You will also want to add it to a warm bath and diffuse throughout the room.

547. Moles:

You can get rid of moles by putting a drop of frankincense oil directly on the mole multiple times throughout the day.

548. MRSA:

To be able to get relief from MRSA you can massage the frankincense oil into the pads of your feet and across your chest. It is also a good idea to use a diffuser in your home or to inhale through a steam tent as long as it does not seem to aggravate or worsen the condition.

549. Multiple Sclerosis:

To reduce the symptoms of multiple sclerosis you will want to use the frankincense oil on your entire body through a gentle massage. Then you will want to apply to the soles of your feet and diffuse or use a steam tent to inhale.

550. Nasal Polyp:

You can get rid of a nasal polyp by adding one drop of frankincense oil to a steaming pot of water. You can also massage the frankincense oil to the base of your toes.

551. Parkinson's Disease:

To get symptom relief with Parkinson's disease you can inhale frankincense oil directly from the bottle or from a steam tent two time each day. You can also have a full body massage with the oil as well as massaging it into the soles of your feet.

552. Postpartum Depression:

Postpartum depression is a very real problem and can be helped with a few drops of frankincense oil to the bathwater or a foot bath. Rub the frankincense oil into your hair or use it during a foot massage. Use the oil as much as you can and inhale from the bottle as much as possible.

553. Prevent Scars:

Adding a drop of frankincense oil to a wound or using during your face care routine will help to prevent scarring. You can also use frankincense to reduce the appearance of scars by putting it directly on the scars.

554. Lipoma Tumors:

You can add two drops of frankincense oil to a steaming pot of water and making a steam tent to inhale until the water is no longer steaming. You should do this daily. You can also massage the oil into your feet using the reflexology points and use it during a full body massage taking care to massage towards the heart.

555. Ulcers:

If you want to cure ulcers you can take frankincense internally in a veggie capsule. Then massage over the area and use with the reflex points of your feet.

556. Nerve Virus:

You can massage frankincense all over your body moving towards the heart or massage the oil into the reflexology points on your feet if you have a nerve virus. You can also add the oil to your bath water.

557. Warts:

Frankincense oil can help warts go away quickly if it is applied directly to the wart each day.

558. Wrinkles:

Another great use for frankincense oil is to help get rid of wrinkles. You can do this by gently massaging the oil into the skin in upward motions each day.

559. Other Uses:

There are so many other uses for frankincense oil. One thing that it does that is unique is that it can penetrate the blood-brain barrier. This means that is great for reversing the signs of aging, healing insect bites, carbuncles, diphtheria, respiratory illnesses, respiratory diseases, healing, gonorrhea, high blood pressure, headaches, herpes, laryngitis, hemorrhaging, jaundice, wounds, pituitary gland functions, pineal gland functions, keeping infections away, sciatic pain, tonsillitis, snake bites, tension, sores, syphilis, spiritual awareness, pneumonia, nervous conditions, stress, prostate issues, and meningitis.

Tumeric Oil Uses

For Health and Healing

560. Inflammation:

Tumeric oil is known as a great anti-inflammatory. This means that it is great to help relieve pain and inflammation. You can use it in combination with frankincense for a number of different types of inflation or alone to treat skin inflammation.

561. Arthritis:

One of the most painful conditions that someone might experience is arthritis. This is something that tumeric oil can be very beneficial for as it helps to speed up the arthritic healing time. It can also help to prevent arthritis. Getting a massage over the joints with the use of tumeric oil is one way to stay healthy and to help reduce the amount of joint pain that you feel.

562. Cancer Shield:

Tumeric oil can work as a cancer shield. Cancer grows in your body constantly through the years. Not all people develop cancer but sadly more people are finding that they are developing cancer in recent years. One of the things that you can do is use tumeric oil to fight the free radicals that are in your body that can cause cancer.

563. Digestion:

If you have stomach problems you can use tumeric oil for a number of benefits. The compounds are on known to play a major role in digestion and can help with digestive issues. They can also help to reduce gas and help prevent the formation of gas. Plus you can use tumeric oil to reduce constipation and to help with regularity.

564. Acne:Many

Young people suffer from acne. Tumeric oil is a great antiseptic that helps with treating acne. You can apply it over your entire face to help detoxify skin and keep it cleaner. All you have to do is apply the oil directly to your face and gently massage. Then you can gently wash it off with soap after thirty minutes. This will help to rejuvenate your skin and remove impurities.

565. Scalp Health:

Tumeric oil can also help you to have a healthy scalp and treat common problems that you might have like dandruff. You can take a few drops of tumeric oil and massage it directly onto your scalp and then let set for 15 minutes. You can rinse and shampoo as usual after that time.

566. Sprains:

You can use tumeric oil to treat painful sprains. You can use a gentle massage with the tumeric oil and it will help to treat sprains and eliminate the pain that they cause. It also works as an anti-inflammatory.

567. Industrial:

The food industry has used tumeric oil as a spice. In the pharmaceutical industry it has been used in anti-microbial, anti-inflammatory, antiseptic, pain relief, anti-fungal, and in ointments.

568. Liver:

Tumeric oil helps to support healthy liver function and can keep your liver healthy.

569. Other Benefits:

There are many other benefits to the use of tumeric oil. They include being an antibacterial, anti-allergen, anti-parasitic, anti-fungal, anti-worm, anti-venom, and antiviral. You can use tumeric oil to treat a number of conditions and ailments.

IN YOUR HOME

570. Environmental Protection:

You can use tumeric oil to protect yourself and the environment around you. It can help to make the air cleaner. All you have to do is add a few drops to the vaporizer, mix with potpourri, or put it in your diffuser. It will help to kill the microorganisms that are actually in the air which will keep your environment healthy.

MYRRH OIL USES

FOR HEALTH AND HEALING

571.   Respiratory System:

There are a lot of benefits for your respiratory system with the use of myrrh oil. You can use myrrh oil as a medication to help cure many respiratory illnesses like the common cold, bronchitis, sore throats, coughs, and asthma. It also has astringent properties that are known for getting rid of phlegm and stopping runny noses. You can also help get rid of respiratory congestion and boost functions of the respiratory system.

572.   Digestive System:

There are many things that you can do with myrrh oil and the digestive system. It helps with enhancing the flow of the digestive juices and helping with food absorption. This will help to stop problems with gas, stomach aches, diarrhea, stomach spasms, dyspepsia, and indigestion. You can also use myrrh oil to clean and remove toxins from the digestive tract.

573.   Blood Circulation:

You can increase blood flow to all of your body parts with the use of myrrh oil. When the blood is drawn to the skin's surface it helps to promote oxygen and nutrients to all of the different parts of the body. This will help with functioning in all of the body parts while helping you to have optimum health.

574.   Wounds:

You can promote wound healing with myrrh oil. You can use the oil as an astringent, analgesic, and antiseptic so it does well with helping to heal wounds quickly. It can also help to increase the number of white blood cells that your body produces. It helps with gastric ulcers, skin injuries, and all other types of wounds.

575.   Skin:

Your skin can benefit greatly from myrrh oil. Myrrh oil uses an increase in the blood circulation to help with a number of different ailments like skin ulcers, wrinkles, tissue degeneration, skin infections, chapped skin, and blemishes. It can soothe and calm the skin while helping to make the skin softer and smoother and restoring youth.

576.   Hair:

Myrrh oil can also work great when used to clean the scalp because it will help to increase the amount of nutrients that flow from the scalp into your hair. It will also help to deeply moisturize your hair. The anti-fungal properties that are found in myrrh oil help with hair conditions that include hair loss and dandruff.

577.   Teeth:

If you are trying to improve your dental health then myrrh oil is a great choice for you. You can often find myrrh oil in toothpastes, gum creams, and mouthwashes. It works great to treat spongy gums, gum inflammation, mouth ulcers, sore throats, loosening of teeth, and gingivitis.

578.   Immune System:

Using myrrh oil is a great way to boost the immune system. It helps to boost the function of the white blood cells while increasing the production. You can fight a number of different types of body infections, heal the digestive tract, lower body temperature during a fever, stimulate appetite during illness, and reduce stomach disorders.

579.   Emotional Bonding:

There are many emotional benefits to using myrrh oil. You will be able to create stronger bonds with other people and will be able to have stronger emotional bonds. Using myrrh oil can help you to increase your level of trust as well as well as make you feel more secure and like you belong.

580. Spirituality:

Myrrh oil will help you to have a direct path between your soul, mind, and body. It stimulates the emotions controlling the brain. This will help you to reduce the amount of feelings that you have associated with depression, restlessness, insecurity, apathy, weakness, and rejection. You will be able to increase your spiritual wellness and connection with the use of myrrh oil. It will also help to block the negative energy that is trying to make its way into the body while creating a calm and peaceful atmosphere to promote self awareness.

581. Feelings of Abandonment:

You can diffuse the myrrh oil or put one or two drops of myrrh oil in your palms and then cup over your nose and mouth while you breathe naturally.

582. Brain:

You can keep your brain healthy by massaging three or four drops of myrrh oil onto the back of your neck and your forehead. Make sure that you are working the oils into the reflexology points on your feet and/or that you are taking internally in a veggie capsule. You can also mix myrrh with frankincense, Hawaiian sandalwood, lavender, and sandalwood to make a brain boosting blend that is perfect for times when you are studying or trying to learn.

583. Cancer:

If you are worried about cancer in a specific area of your body you can massage three or four drops of myrrh oil onto the area. You can also work the oil into the reflex points that are on your feet. In addition myrrh oil can be taken in a veggie capsule for helping with cancer. You can also use the blend that is discussed above when talking about the brain health.

584.   Congestion:

You can massage myrrh oil into your chest, neck and throat to help you with congestion. This can be repeated throughout the day.

585.   Connecting:

When you are using myrrh oil it will help you with your ability to connect to those around you. You can diffuse the myrrh oil throughout the room that you are in during social gatherings to increase your ability to connect with others. You can also put one or two drops in the palms of your hand to cup around your nose and mouth while breathing.

586.   Dysentery:

If you are suffering from dysentery you can put several drops of myrrh oil on your stomach or the bottom of your feet. This can be done several times a day and myrrh oil can be layered with lemon oil or eucalyptus oil.

587.   Fear:

If you are fearful you can diffuse the myrrh oil. You can also put one or two drops of the oil in your hands and cup them over your nose and mouth. Then you just breathe naturally to get the benefits of this mood altering oil.

588.   Gum Disease:

If you suffer from gum disease you can find healing benefits from the myrrh oil. Just add one or two drops of the oil to your toothbrush each time that you brush. You might want to combine the myrrh oil with clove oil as the combination has been shown to be beneficial to many different aspects of oral health including the gums and mouth.

589. Hashimoto's:

Anyone suffering from Hashimoto's will find that they can get relief from diffusing myrrh oil into the room that they are in. They can also find relief by inhaling a few drops that have been put on their hands. Plus you can put the myrrh oil on top of the area where the thyroid is This can be layered with lemongrass for additional benefits.

590. Hepatitis:

Hepatitis is a devastating condition and you can easily find relief by diffusing myrrh oil or inhaling it from your hands. Additionally you can apply a few drops to the soles of your feet and over your liver multiple times each day. If you are suffering from hepatitis you can blend it with frankincense, melaleuca, and any additional antiviral essential oils.

591. Hyperthyroidism:

If you suffer from hyperthyroidism you can inhale myrrh oil from your hands throughout the day or you can diffuse. You can also apply it over your thyroid and then layer with lemongrass for additional benefits.

592. Infections:

There are many different uses for myrrh oil with infections. You can use it as a topical agent, an aromatic, or internally. You can also mix the myrrh oil with oregano oil for some additional benefits.

593. Feelings of Insecurity:

If you struggle with feelings of insecurity then you can apply several drops of the myrrh oil topically to your pulse points, temples, or the back of your neck. You can diffuse the oil or you can put a few drops in your hands and then cup them around your mouth and nose and breathe slowly and deeply.

594.   Liver Cirrhosis:

If you suffer from cirrhosis of the liver you can massage three or four drops of the myrrh oil over the area where your liver is at. You can also use that for a natural detox or with frankincense to improve your liver health.

595.   Pain Relief:

You can get pain relief with myrrh oil by massaging a few drops into the area where you are experiencing pain. You can layer the oils with frankincense or with multiple oils to form a muscle or joint blend or a tension blend.

596.   Parasites:

If you are suffering from issues concerning parasites you will be able to add five or six drops of the myrrh essential oil to a veggie capsule to take internally between one and three times each day. You can also add in oregano oil to help boost the power to fight the parasite.

597.   Prostate Cancer:

Myrrh oil is known to help fight against prostate cancer. You can put five or six drops of the oil into a veggie capsule. You then take the capsule internally with food between two and three times each day. You can also apply the myrrh oil topically to the area where the prostate is at.

598.   Sunburns:

To quickly heal sunburns and relieve the pain that they cause you can add one or two drops of myrrh oil, one or two drops of lavender oil, and one or two drops of helichrysum to a base that has been made from coconut oil or aloe vera gel. You can apply this to skin immediately after your skin has been exposed to the harmful rays of the sun.

599.   Sun Protection:

You can add several drops of myrrh oil to your skin to be able to offer it sun protection. You can also use myrrh oil in homemade sunscreen.

600. Thyroid:

You can help to support your thyroid function by diffusing myrrh oil in your room. You can also apply several drops topically to the thyroid or you can inhale from your hands or even directly from the bottle.

601. Feelings of Trust:

You can improve your ability to trust someone by diffusing myrrh oil into the room. You can also add one or two drops of the myrrh oil to your palms to cup over you mouth and nose and inhale naturally.

602. Tumors:

Myrrh oil can help you to get rid of tumors. You can do this by rubbing three or four drops of the oil over the area where the tumor is at and by rubbing the oil into the reflex points on the feet. This will help to speed up the body's natural ability to heal.

603. Duodenal Ulcers:

If you are suffering from a painful duodenal ulcer then you can take myrrh oil internally to help heal it. You can put two or three drops of the myrrh oil into a veggie capsule to be taken with food. You can take these up to three times each day.

604. Skin Ulcers:

Myrrh oil can also be used to help treat skin ulcers. You just need to put anywhere from one to three drops of the myrrh oil to the ulcer and the surrounding areas of the skin. You will be able to repeat this as desired.

605. Vaginal Infections:

If you have a vaginal infection you can put two drops of the myrrh oil on a tampon and insert it for 30 minutes. You can also apply two drops topically. Finally you can massage the reflexology points on the feet between one and three times each day while using the myrrh oil.

FOR BEAUTY

606.   Chapped or Cracked Skin:

It is easy to heal chapped and cracked skin when you mix together one teaspoon of coconut oil with two or three drops of myrrh oil and apply it to the area where the skin is cracked or chapped.

607.   Stretch Marks:

One of the best things that you can do for stretch marks is to massage two or three drops of the myrrh oil over the stretch mark each day. You can prevent stretch marks by mixing myrrh oil with coconut oil and using this on the skin two to three times daily during pregnancy or other times when stretch marks are likely.

Conclusion

Thank you again for downloading this book!

I hope this book was able to inspire you to start to use essential oils.

Essential oils offer a number of healing benefits that can help you in multiple areas of your life. You will find that with regular essential oil use that you are healthier and that you have a stronger immune system.

Good Luck!

DID YOU ENJOY THIS BOOK?

I want to give big thanks to my readers who have purchased and read this book. I am much thankful to all my clients for giving me such an honor.

Can I ask you guys for a quick favor though?

If you have really enjoyed reading this book and if you have earned some great knowledge then please let me know by feedback.

Click Here.

Feedback and your responses are very important for me. I will read all your comments and I will really appreciate them. Soon I will be up with more books for you. Till then have a good bye!

Thanks so much.

Samantha K. Ray

DO YOU WANT FREE BOOKS?

Receive free books directly to your inbox!

We promote our new books and give them for free for the first 5 days of publication.

We publish up to 5 books per week, in various topics like food, health, parenting, personal finance, etc.

Click here to start receiving your free books.

Thank you and good luck!

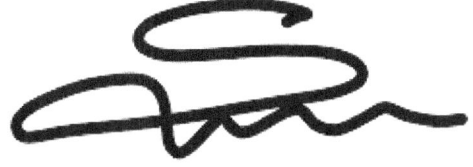

Samantha K. Ray

www.ingramcontent.com/pod-product-compliance
Lightning Source LLC
Chambersburg PA
CBHW081220280526
45787CB00006B/2461